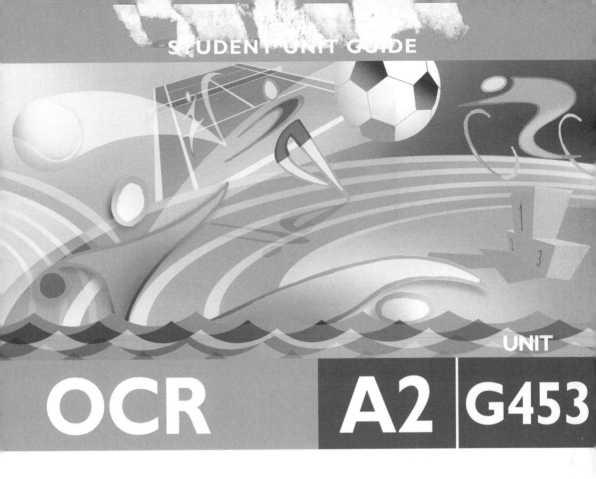

OCR | **A2** | UNIT **G453**

Physical Education

Principles and Concepts across Different Areas of Physical Education

Symond Burrows, ng and
Michaela

I0682643

9 12000063624

Philip Allan Updates, an imprint of Hodder Education, an Hachette UK company, Market Place, Deddington, Oxfordshire OX15 0SE

Orders

Bookpoint Ltd, 130 Milton Park, Abingdon, Oxfordshire OX14 4SB
tel: 01235 827720
fax: 01235 400454
e-mail: uk.orders@bookpoint.co.uk

Lines are open 9.00 a.m.–5.00 p.m., Monday to Saturday, with a 24-hour message answering service. You can also order through the Philip Allan Updates website: www.philipallan.co.uk

First printed 2010

Impression number 5 4 3 2 1

Year 2014 2013 2012 2011 2010

This guide has been written specifically to support students preparing for the OCR A2 Physical Education Unit G453 examination. The content has been neither approved nor endorsed by OCR and remains the sole responsibility of the authors.

Printed by MPG Books, Bodmin

Hachette UK's policy is to use papers that are natural, renewable and recyclable products and made from wood grown in sustainable forests. The logging and manufacturing processes are expected to conform to the environmental regulations of the country of origin.

Contents

Introduction

■ ■ ■

Content Guidance

■ ■ ■

Questions and Answers

Introduction

About this guide

This unit guide is written to help you prepare for **Unit G453: Principles and Concepts across Different Areas of Physical Education**. There are three sections to this guide:

- Introduction — this provides advice on how to use the unit guide, an explanation of the skills required for Unit G453 and suggestions for effective revision.
- Content Guidance — this summarises the specification content of Unit G453.
- Questions and Answers — this provides examples of questions from various topic areas, together with student answers and examiner comments on how these could have been improved.

The specification

The specification describes the topics that you need to learn for Unit G453. Study it closely. If you do not have a copy of the specification, either ask your teacher for one or download it from the OCR website: **www.ocr.org.uk**

The specification for Unit G453 is divided into five options. Section A comprises the sociocultural options:

- Historical studies
- Comparative studies

Section B contains the scientific options:

- Sports psychology
- Biomechanics
- Exercise and sport physiology

You have to study three options including at least one from Section A.

In addition to describing the content of the unit (which sometimes provides detail that could earn you marks), the specification gives information about the unit tests. It also provides information about other skills required in Unit G453. For example, you need to develop the skills of interpreting and drawing graphs and diagrams.

You may find it useful to read the examiners' reports from previous exams as they become available, and to look at relevant past papers and mark schemes. These show the depth of knowledge examiners are looking for, as well as pointing out common student errors and providing advice on how to avoid these so you can achieve a better grade.

Study skills and revision strategies

Effective study skills and revision strategies are an important part of ensuring success in your A-level PE exam.

Organising your notes

As an A-level PE student you will accumulate lots of notes, diagrams, past-paper questions and so on. Keep such information in an organised manner. For revision, you should make your notes clear and concise. You could organise them under main headings and sub-headings with key points highlighted or in italics. Numbered lists are useful in the presentation of material, as are tables and simple diagrams.

After lessons, check your understanding of your notes and read them through. If they are unclear, ask a friend for advice or ask your teacher for further explanation.

Organising your time

Make a revision timetable to ensure you use your time effectively. This should allow enough time to cover *all* the specification content. Your revision timetable should be realistic and fit around other demands on your time. Revision sessions that last longer than an hour can be counter-productive, so allow for short relaxation breaks. By writing up revision notes on cue cards or postcards you can easily revise small pieces of information in short bursts, for example on journeys to school or college.

Revision strategies

To revise a topic well, you should work carefully through your notes, using a copy of the specification to make sure everything is covered. Summarise your notes down to key points in each topic area. Topic cue cards that summarise key facts and give visual representations of the material can be useful.

In many ways, you should prepare for a unit test like an athlete prepares for a major event. An athlete trains every day for weeks or months beforehand, practising the required skills in order to achieve the best result on the day. So it is with exam preparation: everything you do should contribute positively to your chances of doing well in the G453 paper.

The following points summarise some possible strategies you may wish to use:
- Create a revision timetable.
- Spend time revising in a quiet room, sitting upright at a desk or table with no distraction (turn off your television, mobile etc.)
- Regularly test yourself on topics revised to see how well you know them. (NB Revise what you don't know as well as what is already understood; avoiding difficult areas is not the best way of preparing for the exam.)

- Do some past-paper questions in all topic areas to highlight gaps in your knowledge and improve your exam technique.
- Spend some time doing 'active revision' (e.g. in discussion with friends studying PE, reading the sports pages, watching the news and sports programmes, summarising notes and writing your own cue cards).

The unit test

The Unit G453 test is divided into two sections that follow the order of the specification topics listed above. You need to answer three questions in total, including at least one from Section A (the Historical and Comparative options).

In the exam, each topic begins with a number of structured questions with clearly defined mark allocations, normally 4–6 marks. In all, these questions are worth 15 marks. The final part of each question will be a 'levels' question worth 20 marks. The criteria applied by examiners to determine these levels include the quality of your written communication and the number of relevant points you make. You are trying to gain as many as possible of the 105 available marks in the 2½-hour time limit. Your performance will count for 35% of your whole A-level.

In the exam, it is important to write clearly in the spaces provided within the answer booklet. Avoid writing anything that you want marked in the margins — the margins may be lost if papers are scanned for online marking.

Questions may have some words emphasised (e.g. in bold type). This is to draw your attention to key words or phrases that you need to consider in order to answer the question as well as possible. These include:
- Define — give a clear, concise statement or meaning of a word or term.
- Explain — give an answer with reasons to justify it.
- Describe — give an accurate account of the main points in relation to a task set.
- Critically analyse/evaluate/discuss — put both sides of an argument or debate, stating your opinions as appropriate.
- State/give/list/identify — show understanding of unique or key characteristics.
- Apply/demonstrate knowledge — use practical sporting examples to illustrate your understanding of theoretical content.
- Characteristics — features or key distinguishing qualities.
- Benefits — positive outcomes.

Further useful guidance on answering Unit G453 exam questions is provided in the Questions and Answers section of this guide.

The day of the exam

Allow plenty of time and arrive punctually so you are as relaxed as possible.

As you work through the paper, read each question at least twice, highlighting key words or phrases on which to focus your answer. Make sure your writing is legible.

Content
Guidance

Unit G453 is made up of two sections. Section A comprises two options on the sociocultural aspects of PE: **Historical studies** and **Comparative studies**. Section B comprises three options on the scientific issues: **Sports psychology**, **Biomechanics**, and **Exercise and sport physiology**. You have to study three options including at least one from Section A.

Each subject is explored in the context of its impact on participation and performance in physical activity as part of a balanced, active and healthy lifestyle.

This Content Guidance section summarises the key information you need to understand and apply in the G453 unit test. It also includes useful hints on 'What the examiner will expect you to be able to do'. You must read other texts and use other resources to achieve a full understanding of the topics covered in the specification. Make sure that you can give relevant sporting examples for all topics.

Option A1: Historical studies

Popular recreation in pre-industrial Britain

Overview of sport before 1800

Before 1800, the population of the UK was almost totally rural. There were two main groups:
- The gentry had time and the economic and social advantages to pursue activities such as real tennis, which reflected their superior position in society.
- Peasants only had time to play sport on holidays or 'holy days'. They had less access to resources and travel, so their activity was localised and used ready-to-hand materials.

Social and cultural determinants of popular recreation characteristics

Until the latter part of the nineteenth century, the activities of most people were influenced by a number of social and cultural factors:
- natural — used existing facilities
- occasional — limited free time/religious constraints
- played on festivals/holy days — limited free time, pagan/religious origin of activities, e.g. Shrove Tuesday
- rural — most people lived in small market towns
- cruel/violent — harsh society
- local versions — limited travel/communication
- simple unwritten rules — the peasant population was illiterate
- wagering — betting was always part of these activities

Case study activities

Popular recreation activity	Impact on the upper classes/gentry	Impact on the lower classes/peasants
Bathing and swimming	Increased skills and general health and fitness	Mainly hygiene benefits
Athletics	Developed skills and improved health and fitness	As for the upper classes, but pedestrianism for the lower classes
Football	The mob version was frowned on so had limited impact	Force, not skill, was important; lots of injuries resulted

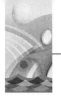

Popular recreation activity	Impact on the upper classes/ gentry	Impact on the lower classes/ peasants
Cricket	Increased skills and general wellbeing as an outdoor summer game	As for the upper classes
Real tennis	Skill development, health and fitness	None (played only by the upper class)

Characteristics of early bathing and swimming

This reflected the characteristics of popular recreation because it was:

- Natural — people could bathe and swim in ponds, lakes and rivers.
- Simple — there were few rules; bathing and swimming was mostly for cleanliness, safety and fun. It was unusual to have competitions at this time.
- Occasional — mostly in the summer season.
- Mainly rural — but some unpolluted urban rivers were also used as time went on.
- Class divided — both classes would bathe/swim, but the social classes did not mix.

Characteristics of athletics and pedestrianism

Simple and cheap	Racing on foot — running or walking
Festival	Popular as a spectacle for the public — exciting contests were associated with events (e.g. prize fighting)
Wagering	Wagering (betting) was encouraged in the crowd — it involved prize money, which sometimes led to cheating/match fixing
Courtly	A challenge to the gentleman amateur — test of courage and fitness
Patronage	Represented earnings or an occupation for the professional/lower-class walker or runner as it was 'patronised' by gentry
Occasional	Major competitions were occasional or special events
Rules	'Challenge rules' were established by competitors/organisers

Characteristics of mob games

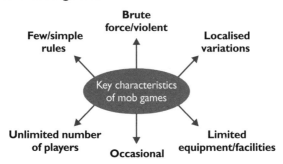

Characteristics of cricket as a popular recreation

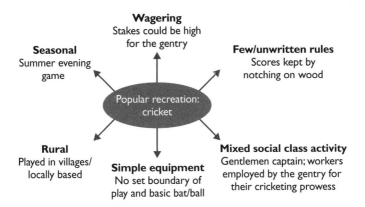

Characteristics of real tennis

Real tennis was an exclusive activity, restricted to the gentry. Its characteristics represent the epitome of rational sport, 400 years before the rational movement evolved in the mid-nineteenth century.

Courtly	Restricted to the aristocracy and royalty — acts of law forbade servants and labourers from playing. Expensive due to the facilities and equipment required
Geographically widespread	Spread throughout the country in castles, fine houses and gentlemen's clubs in towns
Rules	Sophisticated and complex codification. Written rules with specialist language. Literacy necessary to understand these. Dress code and regulations for spectators, who were separated from players
Etiquette/non-violence	Respectable code of behaviour. Skilful not forceful — tactics and strategies required
Regular, leisure pursuit	Played regularly as 'leisured classes' had plenty of free time
Specialist facilities	Purpose-built facilities required

How the case study activities link to modern-day participation

- Swimming — lake-based swimming clubs still exist with an emphasis on swimming for health, fitness, safety and survival purposes.
- Athletics — 'athletic' pursuits continue as part of annual rural sporting contests (e.g. Much Wenlock Games).
- Football — 'mob football' continues in traditional annual events (e.g. Haxey Hood and Ashbourne mob games).
- Cricket — this continues as a game encouraged in all social classes as an active summer pursuit.

- Tennis — in its 'real tennis' format it continues as a game linked to the upper classes in society.

What the examiner will expect you to be able to do

- Describe key characteristics of popular recreation.
- Explain the social and cultural factors that influenced the nature and development of popular recreation activities in pre-industrial Britain and their impact on the physical skills/health and fitness of participants at the time.
- Describe the varying opportunities for participation between the peasants and gentry in a two-tier society.
- Analyse the following case study activities as popular recreation and in terms of their impact on modern day participation: bathing and swimming, athletics, football, cricket and tennis.

Rational recreation in post-industrial Britain

As society developed following urbanisation and the Industrial Revolution, sport became more **rational**. It was played regularly, to set rules, in purpose-built facilities. There was an ethos of fair play, and gambling was controlled. Elements of both amateurism and professionalism were evident as sport became rationalised.

Rational recreation and popular recreation characteristics

Rational recreation	Popular recreation
Regular competitions, held regionally, nationally and internationally	Occasional events and competitions held locally
Strict codification	Simple, unwritten rules
Respectable, fair play, non-violent	Violent, unruly, cruel
Control of gambling	Wagering
Purpose-built facilities	Natural and simple environment
Urban	Rural
Skill based, tactical	Strength based with few tactics

Tip You need to know the characteristics of rational recreation and understand the cultural and societal factors that influenced them.

Influence of the Industrial Revolution on the development of rational sport

First half of the nineteenth century (negative effects):

- Migration of the lower classes into urban areas led to loss of space and overcrowding.
- Lack of time — shift from 'seasonal' to 'machine' time (12-hour days).
- Lack of income — low wages and poverty.
- Poor health — poor working and living conditions, lack of hygiene and little energy to play.
- Loss of rights — restrictions on mob games and blood sports by changes in criminal laws.

Second half of the nineteenth century (positive effects):
- Public provision of baths — health and hygiene improved.
- More time for sport due to the Factory Acts and Saturday half-day.
- Development of the new middle class changed ways of behaving and playing sport — it became more acceptable.
- Influence of ex-public schoolboys via industry, Church etc.
- Values of athleticism spread to the lower classes.
- Industrial patronage led to provision for recreation and sport — factory teams, excursions to the seaside etc.
- Improvements in transport and communication influenced the distances spectators and players could travel, and leagues were established.
- It became cheaper to travel.
- Public provision of parks — people could gather to watch sport (spectatorism).

The transport revolution

The railways increased participation opportunities and spread interest in sport. Faster trains enabled people to travel further and more easily, giving more time for sports matches. Spectators could follow their teams to away matches and regular fixtures developed, creating a need for unified rules or **codification**. Field sports, climbing and walking all became more accessible. Although trains were expensive and used mostly by the middle and upper classes, excursions, often sponsored by employers, allowed working people to travel.

Formation of national governing bodies

Ex-public schoolboys formed many national governing bodies (NGBs) for sport in England during the late 1800s and early 1900s. Codification was needed to ensure sports were played in a uniform manner. Numbers of fixtures and leisure clubs were increasing and these required rules, competitions and leagues. The upper and middle classes wanted to maintain control of sport and preserve their amateur ideals, so professionalism and commercialism had to be controlled.

Case study activities

Bathing/swimming

Spa towns such as Bath and Malvern became popular with the middle and upper classes. River towns developed further, and organised bathing and competitions emerged. Seaside towns grew due to a belief in the therapeutic effects of immersion in water. Improvements in the rail network meant the working classes could visit seaside towns more easily — for example, Blackpool from northern industrial towns.

The Baths and Wash Houses Acts (1846–48) enabled towns to build public baths. The purpose was primarily to promote exercise, combat cholera and fight the spread of disease among the working classes (ultimately increasing efficiency at work). Disease had become widespread due to urban river pollution. The working classes paid 1d to visit the 'second-class facility' in the public baths. The middle classes used the 'first-class facility', consisting of Turkish baths and plunge pools that facilitated competitive races. Amateur clubs and NGBs were established as swimming became a respectable activity. The Amateur Swimming Association (ASA) was formed in 1884.

Athletics
Athletics gradually took on a rational form with the emergence of track and field events.

Upper/middle class	Lower/working class
Sports days — at public schools	Pedestrianism — commercial attraction
Elite athletics clubs — for gentlemen amateurs	Sports days — organised by local promoters in northern industrial towns
Urban athletic sports — a respectable alternative to the old fairs/wakes	Cross-country/harrier clubs — associated with the urban working class

Association football
Rationalised Association football became a game for the masses in late-nineteenth-century Britain.
- It became organised and rule based — NGBs developed, e.g. the FA in 1863.
- It became respectable and accepted — encouraged by the middle classes.
- There were clearly defined roles — for players and officials, e.g. referees.
- Spectators could be accommodated – e.g. stands at grounds.
- Violence was controlled by the laws of the game.
- It was played regularly on a regional and national basis.

The key influences on these developments were:
- improved working conditions:
  - regular and decreasing working hours — e.g. the Saturday half day
  - workers had some spare cash — wages were paid on Saturdays, when matches took place; football was cheap to watch
  - football was seen as a good job to aspire to
- impact of urban expansion:
  - growth of potential spectators — working-class masses in urban areas wanted entertainment
  - limited space — led to reduced or set playing areas (i.e. pitches)
  - the new middle classes saw potential business opportunities in running clubs

- effects of improvements in transport:
  - regular fixtures could be played regionally and nationally — e.g. as a result of railways
  - spectators could travel to matches more easily

Cricket

Characteristics of cricket as a rational recreation activity	How this reflected changes in social conditions
Respectable	Influence of the new middle classes
Roles, structures and codification	Literate and educated classes; NGBs formed
Regular	More leisure time available; improved transport and communications
Local/county/international fixtures	Improved transport and communications aided the development of the professional game
Fair play	Public-school moral emphasis and ethos
Non-violent; gambling controlled	Increased law and order
Amateur versus professional	Britain as a class-based society — unpaid gentlemen amateurs and paid working-class professionals as 'workhorses'
Skilfulness	Increased time to train; employment of specialist coaches

Lawn tennis

Lawn tennis was particularly suitable as a rational activity for the middle classes. They had the necessary space (it was played on the lawns of fine middle-class houses), the organisational experience (for instance from factory ownership) to form private clubs, and the money to provide equipment. The social etiquette surrounding the game allowed respectable, summer social activity and mixing of the sexes.

What the examiner will expect you to be able to do

- Describe the key characteristics of rational recreation and contrast these with the key characteristics of popular recreation.
- Explain how a range of social and cultural factors influenced the nature and development of rationalised sports.
- Explain how the case study activities of swimming, athletics, football, cricket and tennis became rationalised.

The impact of public schools

Nineteenth-century English public schools, such as Eton and Charterhouse, were independent schools of ancient origin. They possessed a number of key characteristics that influenced the development of organised sport and games. They were:

- endowed
- single sex, initially for boys only
- for the gentry
- controlled by trustees
- fee paying
- boarding
- non-local

The Clarendon Report

The 'big nine' public schools were investigated by the Earl of Clarendon in 1864. His report criticised many aspects of public school life and gave advice on how schools could improve. Sport became a key reforming influence in public schools.

Key features of the Clarendon Report
- Public schools were regarded as important for building character. Team games were viewed as a key instrument to achieve this.
- The report discouraged activities that did not promote character building, such as gymnastics and hare and hounds, which were deemed 'less animated' and of little educational value.
- It placed emphasis on moral values as opposed to skilled performance.
- It gave an official justification for the provision of organised physical activity.

The three phases of athleticism in nineteenth-century public schools

Stage 1 1790–1828: boy culture, bullying and brutality
During this period schools were unruly places with a constant battle for control between staff and pupils. Mischief-making and trespass were common.

Key characteristics (What?)
- Institutionalised popular recreation
- 'Melting pot' of experiences brought into schools from all over the country and passed on when boys moved elsewhere
- Some games were adapted, e.g. hare and hounds derived from hunting. Some were adopted, e.g. cricket
- Activities tended to be:
  - violent or barbaric, e.g. mob football
  - childlike, e.g. marbles and hoops
  - based on 'boy culture', e.g. poaching, gambling and drinking
  - based on natural facilities, e.g. exploring the countryside or using the school environment, such as the cloisters at Charterhouse

Social developments (Why?)
- Boarders had the opportunity to play regularly together
- Boys had plenty of free time
- Schools had grounds and space in which to play
- Behaviour of the boys was poor

- Masters had little control outside the classroom
- Sports/games were organised by senior boys who controlled junior boys ('fagging' meant that sixth-formers could bully younger boys)
- There was a **boy culture** of tyranny, chaos, rebellion and violence

Values

- Barbaric discipline: masters 'ruled with the rod' and controlled behaviour through fear (e.g. flogging; the 'thrashing and classics' approach)
- Much resentment between boys and masters
- Schooling was more about contacts (who you know) than education (what you know)
- Sport not encouraged and was seen as time-wasting

Stage 2 1828–42: Dr Thomas Arnold and social control

The early nineteenth century was a time of change in both society and in English public schools. Dr Arnold, headmaster at Rugby School, and other liberal headmasters, wanted to reform public schools so that boys behaved better without the need for severe punishments. Their main aim was to produce Christian gentlemen with high moral behaviour (i.e. **muscular Christianity**). They were against bullying and violence on religious grounds.

Key characteristics (How?)

- Age of reform through liberal headmasters, e.g. Dr Arnold
- Muscular Christianity, i.e. the belief in a strong and fit body to match a robust and healthy soul
- Sixth-form responsibility and social control through prefects
- Games increased in status, regularity and organisation
- Development of house system led to inter-house games such as football and cricket that were believed to develop character

Social developments (Why?)

- Queen Victoria's reign began in 1837: a more civilised society developed, striving for orderliness — 'Victorian values'
- Wild escapades were deemed out of place; boy culture was discouraged
- Laws were passed banning cruelty to animals
- Transport and communications improved (e.g. the Penny Post and railways)

Values

- Muscular Christianity — physical activity for the glory of God, not for its own sake
- Dr Arnold saw social control through games and sport as a way to spread the gospel and produce Christian gentlemen. He wanted to:
  - make punishment by masters less severe
  - make sixth-formers a link between masters and pupils
  - develop the academic curriculum

Stage 3 1842–1914: the 'cult' of athleticism

Athleticism combined physical effort with moral integrity; it involved playing hard but with sportsmanship. By the late nineteenth century, athleticism had reached **cult** proportions. It had become an obsession in many public schools. Team games in particular were valued for their development of character (i.e. the '**games ethic**').

Key characteristics (What?)
- Games now a cult and a source of pride
- Full expression of public-school athleticism
- Academic staff organised daily, compulsory games
- Specialist coaching staff (e.g. Oxbridge 'Blues', who sometimes also played for their schools, or professional cricket coaches)
- 1863–88 — formation of many NGBs
- Emergence of the full structure, kit, equipment and regulations associated with rational sport
- Magnificent facilities, e.g. swimming baths, gymnasia and playing fields
- On-site (e.g. inter-house) and away matches against clubs and schools
- Sports day rivalled speech day for status (sporting success became a means of recruitment)

Social developments (Why?)
- Social control achieved; public schools now respected establishments
- Masters actively supported and promoted sport in school
- 1864: the Clarendon Commission. Other schools and universities copied the 'big nine'
- Emergence of the middle class (the 'industrial aristocracy') led to a growth in the number of middle-class schools (e.g. Clifton and Uppingham) and girls' schools (e.g. Cheltenham Ladies' College)
- Qualities gained through playing games (e.g. leadership, judgement, courage and group loyalty) seen to be beneficial to a career and to the country (1850–70: the era of Britain 'ruling the waves' and expansion of the British empire)

Values
- Cult for masters and boys
- School sport was a vehicle for personal development and the essence of education itself
- The value of games included:
  - moral values (muscular Christianity)
  - encouraging players to 'win gracefully, lose with honour' and 'do your best, give your life'
  - developing commitment, endeavour, brotherhood, fair play, sportsmanship, cooperation and bravery
  - the games ethic — character development through games. Team games (e.g. cricket) deemed to be more valuable than individual activities (e.g. lawn tennis)
- Poaching rejected as a 'barbaric' activity

Why athleticism was delayed in girls' public schools

Tradition
Role of women in society
(girls/women seen as subservient)

Inferiority
Women perceived as
inferior to men and
unable to cope with
exertion of sport

Medical
Participation seen as
harmful to women/girls
(i.e. affecting fertility)

Delay of
athleticism in
girls' public
schools

Social
Sport viewed as
unladylike/unfeminine
(e.g. sweating)

Kit
Concern over
wearing of 'revealing'
clothing for games

Leadership
No female equivalent to boys' headmasters,
who encouraged athleticism

Case study activities

	Stage 1 (1790–1828)	Stage 2 (1828–42)	Stage 3 (1842–1914)
Bathing and swimming	Informal/recreational bathing using available natural resources, e.g. rivers and ponds during summer months	Bathing was more regular and regulated — for the purposes of health, hygiene, safety and recreation	Increased technical development with purpose-built facilities and competitions
Athletics	Informal running and exploration of the countryside, e.g. hare and hounds, with some trespass evident	Trespass less prevalent as it was bad for a school's reputation. Activities such as hare and hounds and steeplechase continued on a more formal, supervised basis	Formalised steeplechase and cross-country running with inter-house sports days as major sporting and social occasions
Football	Played as a mob game — brought from home and adapted to suit each school (e.g. the Eton wall game)	More formalised football rules were set by individual schools. Like other team games, football was played more regularly in the expanding inter-house sporting system	Formalised rules as set by NGBs (e.g. FA, RFU) were used as inter-school fixtures developed. Cult of athleticism led to a craze for team games like football
Cricket	Immediately adopted by public schools as it already had a developed rule structure and upper-class involvement	Like football, cricket played a key part in the expansion of the inter-house sporting competition so had an important role in establishing more social control	Some further technical development with paid coaches, award of 'colours'/caps and regular inter-school fixtures

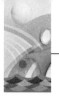

	Stage 1 (1790–1828)	Stage 2 (1828–42)	Stage 3 (1842–1914)
Tennis	Informal ball-and-hand games played against walls/buildings — played as fives or real tennis at this stage of its development	Some fives courts were built although fives remained an informal activity in the main	Fives continued as a recreational pastime. Lawn tennis had developed but was given far more status as a summer game in girls' public schools than in boys' schools

What the examiner will expect you to be able to do

- Describe the characteristics and impact on sporting development of nineteenth-century public schools.
- Demonstrate knowledge and understanding of the Clarendon Report, particularly with respect to its influence on sporting participation.
- Demonstrate knowledge and understanding of the three developmental stages of athleticism in nineteenth-century public schools.
- Demonstrate knowledge and understanding of the reasons for the slower development of athleticism in girls' public schools.
- Explain the impact of nineteenth-century public schools on the development of case study activities (i.e. swimming, athletics, football, rugby, cricket, tennis and other 'striking' games in public schools such as fives, racquets and squash).

Drill, physical training and physical education in state schools

Key terms you must understand

Objectives: the reasons why different syllabuses were introduced and what they were trying to achieve (i.e. the aims).

Content: what was being taught in a lesson.

Methodology: how a lesson was taught and, sometimes, by whom — e.g. **non-commissioned officers** (NCOs) from the services and teachers.

The Model Course (1902)

The main objectives of the Model Course were:
- to increase fitness for military service ('fit to fight')
- to give training in the handling of weapons/weapon familiarity
- to increase discipline and obedience

The main content of the Model Course was:
- military drill
- exercises in unison
- use of staves as mock weapons

The methodology of the Model Course was:
- command–response led by NCOs
- group response — no individuality; pupils were taught in unison in ranks or rows

Reasons why the Model Course was short-lived
The Model Course lasted only 2 years (1902–04). This was because it had no educational focus, did not cater for children's needs and was questionable in its intention of improving the health and fitness of the children. The exercises were mainly static and dull. It was not considered right to treat children as 'little soldiers'.

Syllabuses of physical training (PT)

PT followed on from military drill as teachers and the military profession emphasised the need for young children to experience a balanced set of therapeutic exercises.

Early PT (1904–09)
Developments in this era formed the background to the last PT syllabus (1933). The main objectives of early PT were:
- the therapeutic effects of exercise with emphasis on respiration, circulation and posture (1909 syllabus)
- obedience and discipline
- enjoyment, which started to appear as an aim in lessons
- alertness, decision making and control of mind over body

The main content of early PT:
- was more Swedish in character (1909 syllabus) with recreative aspects to relieve the tedium of former lessons
- introduced dancing steps and simple games

The methodology of early PT:
- 1904 syllabus had 109 tables of exercises for teachers to follow
- 1909 syllabus reduced these to 71 tables
- still formal, still in ranks with marching and 'free-standing' exercises
- unison response to commands continued
- a kinder approach by teachers, with some freedom of choice

The 1919 PT syllabus
The basic objectives of the 1919 syllabus were:
- enjoyment and play for the under-7s
- therapeutic work for the over-7s

This illustrates a key point, namely that age differentiation was starting to appear in the delivery of PT lessons.

The content of the 1919 syllabus:
- involved the same exercises as the 1909 syllabus
- included a special section of games for the under-7s
- stated that not less than half the lesson was to be spent on 'general activity exercises', i.e. active free movement, including small games and dancing

The methodology of the 1919 syllabus allowed:
- more freedom for teachers and pupils
- less formality than previous PT syllabuses

The last PT syllabus (1933)

The industrial depression of the 1930s left many of the working class unemployed; no state benefits were available. The syllabus was viewed as a watershed between the PT syllabuses of the past and the physical education (PE) of the future. This syllabus had one section for the under-11s and one for the over-11s.

The syllabus was influenced by two sources: the **Hadow Report** of 1926 identified the continuing need to differentiate between ages for physical training; and **Dr George Newman** — this was the last syllabus to be published under his direction. Although still set out in a series of 'tables' from which teachers planned their lessons, the syllabus was well respected, detailed and of high quality.

The objectives of the 1933 PT syllabus were:
- physical fitness
- therapeutic results
- good physique/development of posture
- development of mind and body (holistic aims)

The content of the 1933 syllabus:
- athletics, gymnastic and games skills
- group work

The methodology of the 1933 syllabus:
- was set out in tables from which teachers selected
- still used a direct style for the majority of the lesson, mainly from the teachers
- some decentralised parts to the lesson
- group work, and variation of tasks and activities
- encouragement to wear special clothing/kit during lessons
- many schools used the specialist facilities they now had available (e.g. newly built gymnasia)

The development of PE in state schools in the 1950s

The influence of the Second World War

The Second World War saw the destruction of some schools and the growing influence of female teachers as many male teachers enlisted. The apparatus brought into schools following the war was a direct result of wartime commando training. Troops needed to engage in a more mobile style of fighting and to be able to solve problems. The educational value of this type of activity was acknowledged and different styles of teaching emerged in order to develop children more positively, with recognition of their physical, mental, social and emotional needs.

Moving and Growing (1952) and Planning the Programme (1954)

The changes described above were reflected in the publications *Moving and Growing* and *Planning the Programme*, produced by the Education Department. *Moving and Growing* was a guideline for primary schools. Primary school teachers were not trained specifically in PE so needed guidance when planning and delivering it. New apparatus encouraged a problem-solving approach to physical activity. The term 'physical education' had now evolved, giving a different emphasis from the previous 'physical training' by suggesting that the mind needed to be involved as well as the body. This was combined with the movement approach (as advocated by the theorist Rudolf Laban) and led to the following developments in PE teaching:

- exploratory work
- problem solving
- creativity
- skill-based work

PE in the 1950s

The main objectives of PE in the 1950s were:

- to develop physical, social, cognitive and decision-making skills
- to provide a variety of experiences in a fun, enjoyable atmosphere
- to increase involvement for all at their own level of ability

The main content of PE in the 1950s included:

- agility exercises, gymnastics, dance and games skills
- swimming
- movement to music

The methodology of PE in the 1950s:

- was child centred and enjoyment orientated
- was progressive
- involved teachers giving guidance rather than direction
- encouraged problem solving, creativity, exploration and discovery
- encouraged individual interpretation of tasks
- used apparatus in lessons (ropes, bars, boxes, mats etc.)

The start of a 'recreative focus'

In the latter decades of the twentieth century radical changes were made to the physical activities experienced by children at state schools. The (Butler) Education Act of 1944 required local authorities to provide recreational sporting facilities in schools. This was very different from the early-twentieth-century belief that the working classes did not need recreation. Secondary school teachers were now fully trained and therefore no longer depended on a syllabus drawn up centrally. PE teachers were to experience about 40 years of a decentralised system where they had autonomy to choose their own PE programme.

Present-day physical education

National Curriculum PE (1988)

The government introduced the National Curriculum because it wanted:

- more control of education
- more teacher accountability
- national standards to be set for PE
- a wider range of activities to be taught (i.e. more curriculum 'breadth')

This represented a return to a centralised approach to education. All state schools now follow set guidelines about set subjects to teach, and are inspected by Ofsted.

As a result of the Education Reform Act (1988), PE continues to be a compulsory subject that pupils must follow from the ages of 5 to 16. By including it in the National Curriculum, the government evidently considers PE to be an important subject.

The aims of National Curriculum PE in relation to a child's development are to:

- achieve physical competence (i.e. improve physical skills)
- improve self-confidence and knowledge of strengths and weaknesses
- perform in a range of activities
- encourage active use of leisure time
- improve health and fitness
- help children become 'critical performers' (i.e. encourage them to observe and to analyse physical activities knowledgeably)
- learn how to plan, perform and evaluate
- improve cognitive and decision-making skills
- improve social skills and leadership qualities

Has the National Curriculum improved PE in schools?

Yes	No
Uniform experience as a result of the centralised National Curriculum (clear aims and guidelines for teachers to follow)	Less teacher initiative than in the post-war curriculum (e.g. *Moving and Growing*)
Gives wide range of experiences in a variety of activities	Compulsory for ages 5–16, but some groups have relatively low participation (e.g. girls at Key Stage 4)
A variety of roles are experienced (e.g. performer, coach, official)	Limited time available (2 hours a week is the guideline) and PE often has lower status than subjects like maths and science
Preparation for active leisure and lifetime participation	Lack of specialist teachers, equipment and facilities to deliver certain aspects of National Curriculum PE (e.g. outdoor and adventurous activities)

Factors that influence PE/sport provision in schools

A pupil's school PE/sport experience may be positive or negative depending on various factors:

- timetable restrictions — PE may become marginalised, particularly at Key Stage 4 when the demands of GCSE examinations in more academic subjects are high
- lack of funding/resources — for example, schools may find it difficult to fund swimming or outdoor and adventurous activities
- quality of staffing
- quality of facilities
- school–club links can positively influence PE and school sport by improving pupils' access to high-quality coaching, teaching and facilities

What the examiner will expect you to be able to do

- Describe the objectives, content and methodology of the 1902 Model Course, the 1904–33 PT syllabus developments and the *Moving and Growing* and *Planning the Programme* developments in the 1950s.
- Explain the reasons for replacing one approach with another and the effectiveness of such developments on increased involvement for all.
- Explain key developments in PE in the 1970s and 1980s, including a critical evaluation of the impact of National Curriculum PE in state schools.

Option A2: Comparative studies

Sport in the UK

The historical development of sport in the UK

Many UK sports can trace their origins back to the nineteenth century when various key influences were at work in society. One major influence was the public schools, which gave structure and organisation to a number of sports.

Dr Thomas Arnold, headmaster of Rugby School in 1828–42, sought to reform public-school life and improve the behaviour and morals of pupils. He saw organised games as a key vehicle for promoting Christianity and establishing social control.

Sports developed more structure (e.g. rules of play), allowing regular inter-house competitions in football, cricket and so on. As the boys moved on to university, there was a need for widespread agreement on rules so that sport could be played regionally and nationally. In the second half of the nineteenth century, ex-public schoolboys were prominent in the formation of NGBs, which codified many sports.

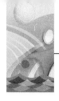

Social class in British society

A strict class system underpinned British society following the Industrial Revolution. Social class affected health, housing and income, as well as the sporting opportunities available as a participant or spectator.

The upper classes had plenty of free time, extensive grounds and money to participate in activity. The newly created middle classes included self-made entrepreneurs aspiring to the upper classes. Both groups could afford to play sport for pleasure, as amateurs, in a spirit of friendly competition. The working classes had little time or money to spend on leisure pursuits. To play sport, they needed payment to compensate for lost earnings. The working classes were therefore associated with professionalism from an early stage in sports such as Association football and rugby league.

Case study: Association football

The historical and cultural influences on changes in the new game of rationalised Association football during the nineteenth century are listed on pp. 14–15.

Case study: rugby football

Rugby football was so popular that the working classes in northern industrial towns adopted the game, but players needed to be paid. The rugby authorities supported the amateur code and opposed payments. Eventually the game split into:

- rugby union — played by amateurs, usually in the south of England
- rugby league — played by professionals from the working classes who took time off work to play

Today, sports need to survive commercially and money enables NGBs to promote the game and finance coaching, competitions and facilities. Rugby union players were being tempted by the professional game and in 1996 the union game turned fully professional.

Geographical determinants of sport in the UK

Geographical factors affect PE and sport in the UK in a number of ways:

- high population density compared with the USA and Australia
- most people live in urban or suburban areas
- potential for mass spectatorism in cities and towns
- well-established transport network enables easy access for participants and spectators
- generally temperate climate — warm summers, cold winters and rain throughout the year
- PE programmes traditionally linked to the seasons (e.g. football, rugby and netball in winter; cricket, rounders and athletics in summer)

Government policy on sports participation

Sports policy in the UK has traditionally been made through a decentralised system (decisions taken at local and regional levels). Until the advent of the National Lottery in the late twentieth century, government funding of sport was relatively low on the agenda. Since London's successful bid to host the 2012 Olympics, government and Lottery funding of sport at all levels has had higher priority. The aim is to finish fourth in the medal table in 2012 and leave a lasting legacy of increased mass participation in sport.

Commercialisation of sport in the UK

The UK has a mixed economy with both public (state) and private (business) sectors. The twenty-first century has seen strengthened links between sport and big business (e.g. football, cricket). Multinational companies compete for exclusive rights to fund high-profile sports, teams and individuals in return for high media exposure. This creates the so-called 'golden triangle' — a mutually beneficial relationship between high-level sport, sponsorship and the media. While minority sports such as netball and hockey miss out, football is cashing in with fame and fortune available to a limited few, particularly in the Premier League.

Social determinants of sport in the UK

In the twenty-first century there are still issues that affect the participation of certain groups, such as the disabled and women, in sport in a negative way:
- reduced opportunity to participate (e.g. through lack of money)
- unsuitable provision (e.g. no access to facilities, clubs and coaches that meet their specific needs)
- low self-esteem (e.g. lack of self-confidence in their ability to take part)

Sporting values

The UK has a long tradition of sporting participation, with many positive outcomes seen to be gained from it, such as:
- Teamwork — developing the ability to work as part of a team through sport/PE.
- Individuality — sports organisations and individuals are free to make their own decisions on participation.
- Fair play — the emphasis on conduct in sport is of great importance at all levels, including in schools.
- Competitiveness versus participation — taking part has traditionally been seen as more important than winning; there is a lack of competitiveness, with less of a 'win ethic' than in the USA.
- Overcoming discrimination — society strives to overcome inequality through sport programmes and initiatives, which often include anti-discrimination schemes (e.g. Kick It Out in football)

PE, school sport and mass participation in the UK

PE programmes in UK schools generally consist of compulsory PE lessons that follow the National Curriculum for pupils between 5 and 16 years. In addition, pupils can choose to participate in **extra-curricular competitive sport** such as inter-house or inter-form competitions within their school or between schools. Such extra-curricular activities have traditionally been at the discretion of teachers. They have varied in quality and quantity due to staff willingness to run them.

The government has introduced a number of initiatives to counter the decline in availability of school sport. These place greater importance on sporting opportunities for pupils (see below).

A strong tradition of team games such as football, rugby and netball continues in extra-curricular sport in UK schools. More recently, as part of the government's health and fitness agenda, more varied extra-curricular programmes have been offered in an attempt to promote lifelong involvement in physical activity.

Health, fitness and obesity levels in young people in the UK
In its report *Tackling Obesities: Future Choices* (2007), the Department of Health predicted that 60% of adults and 30% of children would be classed as obese by 2050.

In 2006 the Information Centre for Health and Social Care published statistics on obesity, physical activity and diet in England. The findings included worrying levels of obesity in young children. The number of children aged 2–15 classified as obese increased from 10.9% in 1995 to 18% in 2005 for boys and from 12% in 1995 to 18.1% in 2005 for girls.

In 2002 figures indicated that a significant number of young people were not active enough. It is clear that health and fitness levels are in decline among young people in the UK and obesity levels are increasing as a consequence of inactivity.

Initiatives promoting PE and school sport in the UK
In the UK, PE and school sport have traditionally been kept apart but there has been a growing awareness of the need to bring them closer together. The **PESSCL** strategy contained a number of sub-programmes to help increase the uptake of sporting opportunities among 5–16 year olds, so that at least 85% experienced a minimum of 2 hours of high-quality PE and school sport each week.

A key aspect of PESSCL was the development of specialist sports colleges. These are secondary schools with a specialist status for sport. They help to deliver the government's targets for school PE and sport. They are designed to provide opportunities for young people and aim to raise standards in PE and sport. They are regional focus points for:
- promoting excellence in PE and sport in the community
- extending links between schools in the community they serve
- helping young people to progress on to careers in sport

PESSCL has developed into PESSYP. Visit the Youth Sport Trust website (**www.youthsporttrust.org**) for more information.

Sport England's new strategy to raise participation was launched in June 2008. Its targets for 2012–13 include:

- 1 million more people doing sport (e.g. through the Sport Unlimited initiative)
- a measurable increase in people's satisfaction with their experience of sport
- playing a key role in the delivery of the Five Hour Sport Offer for children and young people

The pursuit of sporting excellence in the UK

For many aspiring athletes, the opportunity to achieve excellence involves financial support. Financial support tends to come initially from parents, but more formal systems have been established to help aspiring athletes. The Talented Athlete Scholarship Scheme (TASS), World Class Performance Programmes, Lottery funds, sports college scholarships and SportsAid funding are examples.

Aspiring performers also need support such as:
- top-level coaching
- high-quality training facilities
- sport science analysis, support and physiotherapy
- expert advice on personal life and career development

It is important to develop the esteem of elite performers. They must believe they can compete with the best in the world and win. Specialist training camps and elite training groups bring like-minded people together and provide the high-level competitive opportunities necessary to develop the confidence to achieve at the top level.

UK Sport is the key organisation with responsibility for elite sport development in the UK, including for young people. It improves opportunities by funding elite-level athletes via NGBs and its World Class Performance Programme enables performers to devote themselves full time to their sport.

The **UK Sports Institute** (UKSI) network overseen by UK Sport has been important in providing world-class facilities for performers to train and compete in, plus coaches, sports scientists and medical professionals. The UKSI also coordinates research and development, drawing upon best practice from across the world and applying this to UK sports and elite athletes.

Case study activities

The development of cricket, rugby league, rugby union and Association football to their current status is described in *OCR A2 Physical Education*, published by Philip Allan Updates, and elsewhere. Make sure you know how these activities evolved.

What the examiner will expect you to be able to do

- Demonstrate knowledge and understanding of the historical and cultural contexts influencing the development of sport in the UK.
- Demonstrate knowledge and understanding of the determinants of participation in sport, including geography, social aspects, government policy and sporting values.
- Explain how sport, sponsorship and the media in the UK are linked.

- Demonstrate knowledge and understanding of health, fitness and obesity levels among young people and the general population in the UK.
- Demonstrate knowledge and understanding of developments to promote sport in schools and in the wider community.
- Explain opportunity, provision and esteem in the UK in relation to sports excellence.
- Explain how UK Sport and the UKSI contribute to the development of elite performers.
- Explain how cricket, rugby league, rugby union and Association football have evolved to their current status in the twenty-first century.

Sport in the USA

The historical development of sport in the USA

The USA has pursued a policy of isolationism, which has spread into sport. Originally British sports such as cricket and rugby have been rejected because:

- they lack popularity with Americans; for example, Americans do not like the idea of a drawn game, as in cricket
- they lack the dynamic, all-action spectacle that Americans demand when watching sport
- many British sports reflect British middle-class values and traditions, which does not suit the egalitarian, individualist philosophy of Americans

Sports such as cricket and rugby union are at the margins of American society. The 'big four' sports of basketball, American football, baseball and ice hockey are highly promoted and at the forefront. This reflects America's 'new world' culture and its independence as a young, competitive society.

The competitive nature of top-level sport in the USA reflects 'frontierism' and the pioneering spirit of American migration to the West during the nineteenth century.

Geographical determinants of sport in the USA

The USA has a population density of about 70 people per square mile. The majority of people live in urban areas. The densely populated areas have spawned the 'New World' urban sports like American football and basketball.

North America covers a huge geographical range with many climatic zones. The terrain varies from open plain to desert and high mountain ranges, giving many opportunities for outdoor and adventurous activities.

In comparison to the British, Americans are prepared to travel long distances by car. There is an advanced network of interstate highways and urban freeways. Interstate air travel is widely available, and, as in the UK, rail links are well established and played a key role in the early development of structured competitive sport from the late nineteenth century onwards.

Government policy towards sport

At its emergence as an independent nation in the late eighteenth century, the USA founded a new government with a **federal** constitution, effectively creating a republic. As a republic, it has an elected president but, unlike the UK, it has never had a monarchy or privileged class with the power to determine or influence opportunities available. There is also a tradition of self-rule for each state.

A federal constitution means that the powers of government are divided between national and state governments and decentralisation allows power to be distributed throughout the USA. This is reflected in the way education and sport are administered.

Sport and commercialism in the USA

Professional sport is highly organised in America as a commercial industry. The major television companies screen hundreds of hours of sport each day.

The USA is a competitive capitalist society where individual effort and endeavour are desirable characteristics. Capitalism drives both society and sport. For the most successful athletes in the highest-profile sports, the 'golden triangle' means that fame and vast wealth are attainable. For example, in late 2007 the New York Yankees and player Alex Rodriguez agreed a deal for $275 million over 10 years with a multi-million dollar bonus for breaking the home run record.

Social determinants and sporting values in the USA

Ethnicity

Some ethnic groups occupy positions of superiority (for example in terms of economic attainment) and racism towards other 'inferior' groups may result. Racial **discrimination** occurs when these beliefs lead to actions.

Stereotypical views (i.e. negative generalisations) may exist regarding ethnic groups. For example, a stereotypical view of black sports performers is that they are best suited to roles that require physical rather than mental qualities, such as running backs in American football and outfield positions in baseball. A disproportionate concentration of ethnic minority players in certain positions in sports teams is known as '**stacking**'. Stacking can exclude these groups from prestigious or judgement positions. Such pivotal positions are known as 'centrality' positions and require decision-making and leadership qualities that ethnic minorities are stereotypically viewed as not possessing. Stacking is not as prominent in basketball where black players often occupy centrality positions such as point guard.

Ideological influences

As a capitalist, democratic nation, the USA embraces many ideologies (i.e. beliefs, values and attitudes) that influence participation and progression in sport.

Provision of opportunity

In the '**land of opportunity**', success, wealth and happiness are theoretically available to all. The distribution of power in the USA gives the opportunity for free

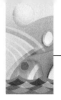

enterprise and reflects individualism. The freedom to seek wealth exemplifies the spirit of the USA.

The 'American Dream' is the belief that happiness is secured through the generation of wealth. It requires hard work, effort and sacrifice to achieve success in this competitive society and failure to win can result in dismissal, e.g. in sport, coaches are often employed on a 'hire and fire' basis.

Pluralistic versus hegemonic culture

There are two main images of US society that you should be aware of.

A **pluralistic society**, in which:
- no one particular group dominates
- each culture retains its own identity and cultural norms
- each culture has the opportunity to influence the operation of the country
- liberty, justice, equality and opportunity are freely available to all cultures and individuals

A **hegemonic society**, in which:
- a single group dominates (i.e. white Anglo-Saxon Protestants — WASPs)
- the dominant group controls the economy and political institutions
- the dominant group uses its influence to shape attitudes, values and cultural norms within society
- other groups become convinced that the dominant group is right and just, which spreads conformity throughout the whole society
- the dominant group tells everyone else that the country lives by and supports the pluralist image

Three sporting ethics

It is also important to understand that three main ethical influences co-exist in American sport and recreation:
- Lombardianism — the Lombardian ethic links to the belief that winning means everything; it is the main motive for participation.
- Counter-culture — this has an anti-competitive focus and emphasises the intrinsic benefits that can be derived from sports participation. An extreme example is 'eco-culture', which involves fun and health promotion in the outdoor environment. The emphasis on participation rather than results is more like the traditional British approach.
- Radical ethic — winning is important as a mark of achievement, but the process of arriving at the achievement is equally important. This ethic prevails in intra-mural college games and is associated with Lifetime Sport, the equivalent of the UK Sports Council's Sport for All.

PE and school sport in the USA

The USA has a tradition of state autonomy, which is reflected in the decentralised education system (each state has control of its own education). The majority of schools do not train students for externally set exams, although some states have introduced a high school 'exit exam'. Completion of studies at high school to a pass standard leads to the award of a high school diploma, which is required for entry to a college degree course.

The concept of a National Curriculum does not exist in the USA. There are a number of core subjects with PE among them. PE programmes are designed and regularly inspected by a superintendent of the local school board. The teacher is required to work through set programmes while assessing student performance.

At high school level, the emphasis is on delivering fitness and direct skill learning. The system allows for variations between schools and ensures that programmes are delivered effectively. There is a framework for progression, but opportunities for 'creative teaching' and counter-culture activities are restricted.

It is important to remember that PE teachers in the USA are separate from sports coaches and generally have lower status.

Decline in participation

Student participation in PE was about 70% in the 1980s but fell below 60% by 2000. The greatest decline comes beyond sixth grade, when pupils progress to junior high school. This decline led to a warning by the National Association for Sport and Physical Education (NASPE) that PE is now seen as an expensive luxury rather than a necessity.

The decline in school PE and consequent disengagement in physical activity has increased concerns about health and fitness levels. Obesity concerns are rising in all affluent countries. Low levels of fitness and obesity in teenagers have been an ongoing issue in the USA since military conscription was made necessary in the Second World War. In 2003, 44 million Americans were registered as obese — an increase of 74% in 10 years.

Strategies are now being introduced to reverse the decline of PE and improve the quality of pupils' timetabled PE experiences, which many, including NASPE, believe are essential for promoting healthy, active lifestyles. Tens of millions of dollars have been invested into a Physical Education for Progress (PEP) programme.

Equality in school PE and sport in the USA

The USA has an active policy of sports provision for different sections of society, particularly for disabled individuals. Federal law states that PE must be provided for students with special needs and disabilities. This provision is called '**adapted physical education**'. It involves diverse programmes that have been modified to enable full participation.

Title IX

Title IX was passed as law in 1972 and is an example of central legislation (i.e. imposed by central government). It addressed the issue of gender equality in all areas of education. In terms of sport, the law was not primarily concerned with opening up traditional male-dominated, physical contact activities like American football to greater female participation. Instead, it focused on widening participation for women in general. Prior to Title IX, opportunities for female inter-scholastic and inter-collegiate sports participation were severely restricted: women experienced segregated and inferior facilities, and women's athletic scholarships were rare.

Title IX has increased standards in women's sports, with raised performance levels in soccer and track and field being celebrated by American society.

Extra-curricular sport in US high schools

In contrast to the provision of daily PE, inter-scholastic sport in the USA is very strong. Most major sports are represented in high schools with an emphasis on American football, basketball and baseball for boys, and track and field, volleyball and soccer for girls. The State High School Athletic Association (SHSAA), a national advisory body with branches in each state, regulates inter-scholastic athletic competition.

Specialist coaches are employed to take charge of school teams and are accountable to the athletic director of the school. They manage both overall PE and inter-scholastic sport. High school sport has high status and interest, with thousands of spectators attending fixtures in high-class facilities. There is a strong tradition of Lombardianism, with coaches being fired if the team is unsuccessful. Players also have a strong motivation to win as college athletic scholarships are on offer.

American ideologies are reflected in inter-scholastic sport — there is opportunity for all to play and excel, but only elite performers achieve athletic scholarships, bringing professional status and the American Dream a step closer.

Summer camps for young people

Several youth agencies such as the YMCA sponsor outdoor activities and some schools offer programmes of 'low-risk' adventure. Outward Bound is an example of a packaged adventure programme that works together with senior high schools to offer wilderness experiences and proficiency courses in outdoor skills and leadership.

Since the mid-twentieth century, the number of summer camps for young people has increased significantly. They take place in the summer holidays and last from a few days to 8 weeks. Most camps have a mission to continue a patriotic culture. For instance, the bugle sounds the morning waking call and the US flag is unfurled and displayed. The children enjoy campfire rituals in the evenings. Such features reflect a military ethos and the spirit of frontierism, both of which underpin national pride.

Mass participation in the USA

The USA is in danger of becoming a spectator rather than a participator society. In 2006 the National Center for Health Statistics stated that just over 30% of adults engaged in regular leisure-time physical activity, meaning that around 70% did not. Only three in ten adult Americans get the recommended amount of physical activity (i.e. 30 minutes' pulse raising/aerobic activity, five times per week). Heart disease is now the leading cause of death among men and women in the USA, and inactivity is a major contributory factor. Obesity is another associated major health issue.

Contemporary initiatives to promote participation

- The President's Challenge is a 6-week programme designed to engage all Americans in making physical activity part of their everyday lives. The challenge includes the Presidential Active Lifestyle Award for performing regular activity beyond the daily goals set for each individual.
- The OneGoal scheme attempts to increase the understanding and awareness of youth ice hockey so it becomes less intimidating to participate and join a club.
- Midnight Basketball Leagues have been set up using outdoor asphalt surfaces with the aim of improving and controlling behaviour, and increasing physical activity among ethnic minorities in particular.

Sport and the pursuit of excellence in the USA

Little Leagues

These cater for 7–16 year olds and form the basis of most American sports. Teams are coached and managed mainly by volunteers such as parents. While there is a strong moral philosophy with an emphasis on safety, the Lombardian ethic is evident from the outset. Specialist coaches are used to raise standards of performance and increase the chances of success. Little League formats reflect the professional game; for instance, mini-Super Bowl finals inspire competition and attract interest from sponsors and the media.

Pathways to professional sport: the college system

Athletic scholarships to US colleges are available for elite high-school performers in most major sports. Athletic associations govern college sports and set the rules governing scholarships. College administrators tend to enrol students who are excellent players but lack academic qualities. Such leniency allows colleges to compete and remain at the highest levels to maintain their commercial viability. The National Collegiate Athletic Association has stated that 20% of football and basketball players enter through such 'special admit' programmes.

Problems in varsity sport occur when coaches, in their quest for success, exert excessive pressure on students and sport loses its value as an educational process. It also becomes an issue when media rights to games are bought and sold, so the academic progress of players becomes less of a consideration than profit.

A scholarship is worth around $10 000 a year, paying for meals, accommodation and tuition fees. The student is then bound by contract to train for long hours and play sport for the college.

Equality and discrimination in American professional sport

Segregation and inequality have featured in organised sport since the nineteenth century. Black players were excluded from Major League baseball until 1947, but since then gradual integration has occurred. To understand such exclusion, you should be aware that American society is organised by wealth and also by race.

WASPs retain domination and make up the controlling hegemonic group. After African-American players broke into white professional sport in the 1950s, a period of 'tokenism' followed. As more black players entered professional sport, they were stacked into positions requiring physical skills, with Anglo-Americans tending to occupy decision-making roles. This centrality endorsed the social order.

The twenty-first century has seen further integration and more even positional distribution. In Major League baseball, 20% of players are black while the National Football League has around 70%. Only about a fifth of players registered with the NBA are white, which represents an exit of Anglo-Americans from the game ('**white flight**').

It appears that the ideologies of freedom and opportunity to pursue the American Dream are becoming increasingly real to women and ethnic minorities in sport. This is reinforced through role models such as the Williams sisters, Tiger Woods and Michael Jordan. Increased self-belief and self-esteem have resulted, with people from ethnic minorities now having the confidence and motivation to strive for recognition in sports, including sports traditionally associated with the dominant white culture group.

Case studies

The main four sports in the USA are American football, basketball, baseball and ice hockey. These sports have become big business and athletes are marketed as assets who can generate funds and advertise products through their skills, showmanship and positive health images. The sports are packaged and presented to the public, often in a brash and energetic style involving huge productions costs — as shows rather than games.

Though these dominant sports possess their own characteristics, they also contain common elements such as high scoring and fast play requiring skill and power. Through the media and sponsors, this creates mass entertainment. The sports businesses are controlled by their owners, and they and their merchandise are heavily marketed. The professional ethos of the Lombardian ethic, with material rewards for success, reflects the US capitalist system discussed earlier.

You need to know and understand how the four main sports in the USA have evolved.

What the examiner will expect you to be able to do

- Explain the historical determinants of sport in the USA that led to the marginalisation of typically British sports and the promotion of the 'big four' sports.
- Explain the current determinants of PE and sport in the USA as they affect opportunities and participation in terms of geography, social aspects, sporting values, and government policy at federal, state and local level.

- Describe the commercialised nature of sport in the capitalist system of the USA.
- Explain the general health, fitness and obesity levels among young people and the general population in the USA.
- Understand the status of and attitudes towards PE in US schools. Give examples of contemporary initiatives promoting PE and sport in schools and the wider community.
- Understand issues relating to equality of opportunity and young people in the USA, particularly in relation to gender and disability. Understand the debates concerning equality and discrimination in the pursuit of excellence.
- Understand the values of outdoor education programmes and the different types available to young people (e.g. summer camps).
- Explain the pathways available to professional sport (e.g. the college system).
- Explain how American football, basketball, baseball and ice hockey originated, evolved and developed into commercialised products in the twenty-first century.

Sport in Australia

Historical, political, social and cultural determinants of Australian sport

Unlike the USA, Australia has maintained close links with its motherland and there is continued evidence of its colonial roots in the education system, sporting ethos and general traditions. The British settlers in Australia readily continued traditional British sports such as cricket and rugby, which gained a firm foothold. This means that sporting relations between the UK and Australia are still close, with regular test series in sports such as cricket, rugby league and rugby union.

System of government

Three levels of government exist:
- central government at a federal level
- six states and two territories — state governments take an active role in promoting sport and PE
- local government in each state — the local level plays an important role in delivering initiatives such as Active Australia to local communities

Australia has a decentralised system of government giving autonomy to each state (i.e. states are self-governing). This means that provision for sport, education, PE and sport in the community is different in each state.

Ideological influences

Twenty-first century Australia desires an inclusive, pluralistic society. Its ideology focuses on being democratic and capitalist, on the Western model. An egalitarian ethos is present. Australia is strongly nationalistic, and sporting success is valued highly by its patriotic population.

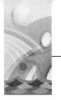
Australia has a reputation for encouraging community participation in all forms of sport. Its favourable climatic conditions support outdoor activities all year round. Australia has over 120 national sports organisations, and around a third of the population are registered as members of sports clubs.

Australia uses sport to try to shed its 'bush culture' image. This culture links to the old frontier values of individuality and ruggedness, which led to male domination and gender discrimination. Such an image does not fit the more egalitarian ethos of twenty-first-century Australia.

Transport, technology and commercialism in sport
Transport systems are well developed with an extensive network of roads along the coast, modern train services and internal air transport systems.

Satellite television has allowed sports coverage from around the world to reach previously remote areas. Australian sports have become increasingly commercialised as sponsors see opportunities to promote their products. Many sports have become professional and new organisations have been set up to cater for them, such as the Australian Football League and the National Soccer League. A number of private sports management companies have emerged, such as the International Management Group (IMG), which secure sponsorship deals, advise on marketing strategies, and negotiate television rights and endorsement contracts.

Geographical determinants affecting PE and sport in Australia

The population of Australia is relatively small and settled largely in and around eight cities. A large percentage of Australia is uninhabitable and the majority of Australians live on low-lying coastal plains around the south and east coast. These have a temperate climate, favourable to outdoor sports. Most people, then, live close to thousands of miles of beach and coastline that provide free and accessible facilities for a range of activities.

PE and school sport in Australia: a case study of Victoria

Following a government examination in the late twentieth century of participation patterns and declining standards of skill and fitness, changes took place in how PE and sport are delivered in Australian schools.

Edith Cowan University in Western Australia presented the **Sport Education and Physical Education Project (SEPEP)** as a model for teaching physical activities. SEPEP provides a framework and is available throughout the Australian PE system but it forms only a small part of curriculum delivery. Teachers are free to adapt it and introduce their own programmes to accommodate variations in student ability, teaching environments and their own expertise. There is no equivalent of the National Curriculum, or Ofsted inspection service in Australia so teachers have professional autonomy.

The state of Victoria set up the **Victoria School Sports Unit** to introduce strategies and ensure that programmes are delivered effectively. PE and sport education programmes are compulsory up to Year 10. The Victoria model has a number of important features such as:

- 100 minutes of compulsory PE each week
- 100 minutes of compulsory sport education each week
- all school teams play in school time

The Victoria School Sports Unit commits to training non-specialist teachers. Courses are intensive and are placed under the all-embracing title of Physical and Sport Education (PASE). All such professional development is financed by government.

Forty schools in Victoria have earned the status of government 'exemplary schools'. Teachers from these schools deliver professional development and share good practice with neighbouring institutions. Grants are given to cover the cost of teacher release and there is considerable prestige associated with such 'exemplary' status.

Victoria is committed to raising the profile of PE and sport. Teachers raise their own profiles as role models by engaging in the Teachers Games (residential sports competitions that give networking opportunities and endorse the participation ethic — the main motive in Australian PE/sports education).

Victoria acknowledges its high achievers in sport with awards for fair play. For example, the de Coubertin awards are presented to students who have made an outstanding contribution to administration, coaching and other roles beyond that of a participant. The award reflects the original spirit of the modern Olympics — that taking part is more important than winning.

Examples of other sport/PE initiatives include:

- The Schools Network
- The Active After-School Communities programme
- The Active Australia/More Active Australia initiative

Outdoor education

Schools generally have good outdoor facilities including playing fields, swimming pools and outdoor gymnasia. Swimming is very popular and has strong emphasis in the school curriculum.

There is a high level of interest in the international Outward Bound movement and the Duke of Edinburgh scheme, but outdoor education for students relies on government support, and staff goodwill and initiative.

There are different types of residential centres in Australia, such as:

- outdoor schools, where students get first-hand experience of the natural environment.
- environmental centres focusing on environmental studies
- outdoor pursuit centres, which provide field centres and opportunities for a wide range of activities

Mass participation in Australia

The **Australian Sports Commission** (ASC) and other government agencies collect information on participation patterns in the 15+ age group via the Exercise, Recreation and Sport Survey (ERASS). In 2006, 66% of people aged 15 and over (i.e. 10.9 million) participated in exercise at least once a week, with 42.8% participating in sport three or more times a week. The most popular activities were walking, fitness activities such as aerobics, and swimming.

The ASC was created following Australia's poor Olympic performance in Montreal in 1976. Its mission is 'to enrich the lives of all Australians through sport'. Its purpose is to administer and fund sport nationally on behalf of the federal government. The ASC is central to an integrated national policy to encourage physical activity at all levels, from mass participation to sports excellence. It works with various national sporting organisations, state and local governments, schools and community organisations to ensure sport is well run and accessible.

The ASC's Strategic Plan 2006–09 set the strategies and framework for meeting its objectives and achieving the outcomes required by government. The 'critical result areas' against which it assesses the implementation of the plan include:
- sustained achievements in high-performance sport by Australian teams and individuals
- maintaining the Australian Institute of Sport (AIS) as a world centre of excellence for the training and development of elite athletes
- the growth in sports participation at grass-roots level, particularly among youngsters, indigenous Australians, women and people with disabilities
- increased opportunities for children to be physically active
- increased adoptions of fair play, self-improvement and achievement

The **More Active Australia** initiative aims to increase participation at grass-roots level. It promotes the social, health and economic benefits of participation.

Sportit! encourages young children to become involved in physical activity. The programme develops basic motor skills used in the major sports of Australia.

The **Modified Sport Programme** adapts adult sports for young children, for example by modifying equipment or rules, as in Netta Netball or Kanga Cricket.

Sport and the pursuit of excellence

The Australian Institute of Sport (AIS)

The AIS is widely acknowledged in Australia and internationally as a world best-practice model for elite athlete development. It is based in the federal capital of Canberra, but decentralised — each state has a replica AIS academy. Each academy currently has its own specialist sports, but they are becoming multi-sport-based. The functions of the AIS are to:
- train top performers in world-class facilities

- give top performers access to high-quality coaches
- undertake sports science research to improve elite-level performances further
- give sports medicine support to get athletes back on track as soon as possible
- provide educational and lifestyle advice to support performers
- use elite performers as role models in sports clubs and schools to inspire others. The Sports Person in Schools Project and AIS Connect programme aim to raise the profile of the AIS and its athletes.

National talent search

The ASC's National Talent Identification and Development (NTID) programme aims to identify and fast-track Australia's next generation of athletes with international medal-winning potential. Between May 2006 and May 2010 the government pledged AU$20 million to support the delivery of NTID initiatives. Such talent identification programmes will help broaden Australia's sporting base and maximise its relatively small talent pool of about 280 000 athletes (compared with 16 million in China and 1.2 million in the UK).

The draft system: a pathway to professional sport

A 'draft' process is used in the USA and Australia to allocate certain players to sports teams. Teams take it in turns to select from a pool of eligible players. When a team selects a player, it receives exclusive rights to sign that player to a contract.

The best-known type of draft is the 'entry draft', used for players who have recently become eligible to play in a league. Depending on the sport, the players may come from college, high school or junior teams. An entry draft prevents bidding wars for young talent and ensures that no single team can take all the best talent. Poorly performing teams from the previous season usually choose first in the post-season draft. This happens in the Australian Football League Draft — the annual draft of new unsigned players by Australian Rules football ('Aussie Rules') teams. Here, clubs receive 'picks' based on the position in which they finish during the season.

Equality and discrimination in Australian sport

Sport and gender

Early colonialist attitudes led to discrimination towards women in society: a flourishing masculine culture restricted women to 'parlour games'. In the mid-twentieth century female sports performers began to emerge in athletics and swimming for instance, but even then, female performers were deemed 'too masculine' if they exhibited too much aggression or competitiveness, and often had their sexuality challenged.

The second half of the twentieth century saw a gradual change in attitudes, with women successfully competing in a wide range of activities. Yet in a country where women are in the majority, sports representation is still disappointingly low.

In 1984, the Commonwealth Sex Discrimination Act was passed, followed by several state equal opportunity Acts, making it unlawful to discriminate against a person on the grounds of sex, marital status or pregnancy. Sports clubs were forced to offer women full membership.

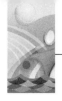

Australia recognises the need to develop equality, for instance via mixed-sex school PE programmes and the use of female role models in clubs and schools. The Women and Sport Unit of the ASC is developing policies that address gender issues in sport to improve participation and the success of female elite performers.

Disability sport in Australia

Sports CONNECT helps people with disabilities to become active in sport and recreation in whatever roles they choose. It helps disability groups understand the benefits of sport and aims to increase participation by ensuring that links between sports and disability groups are effective.

Paralympic sport in Australia is gaining prominence. The Australian Broadcasting Corporation (ABC) and the Australian Paralympic Committee (APC) announced a collaboration to bring the 2008 Paralympics into every household in Australia and ABC television broadcast more than 100 hours of coverage. APC president Greg Hartung said it was fitting that Australia's largest-ever 'away team' of 170 athletes and 123 officials received the most extensive Paralympic Games coverage by a television network in the world.

Case studies

The case study activities for sport in Australia are cricket, rugby league and rugby union, Association football and Australian Rules football. You must learn how these sports have evolved.

What the examiner will expect you to be able to do

- Understand the historical and cultural factors affecting participation in Australia, particularly those linked to the concept of the UK as Australia's 'motherland'.
- Understand the factors affecting opportunities for PE and sport in Australia concerning geography, social aspects, government policy and sporting values.
- Understand how sport in Australia has become commercialised.
- Demonstrate knowledge and understanding of sport participation levels among the whole population and, in particular, among young people in Victoria.
- Outline how projects are increasing participation and encouraging involvement in sport and outdoor activity both in schools and the wider community (e.g. SEPEP, PASE and More Active Australia). Explain the role of the ASC.
- Explain the impact of the environment on outdoor education in Australian schools.
- Understand the structure and functions of the AIS and national strategies to encourage excellence.
- Explain how cricket, rugby league, rugby union, Association football and Australian Rules football have originated and developed.

Option B1: Sports psychology

Individual influences on the sports performer

Personality

Personality is defined as the unique psychological and temperamental features of an individual.

Trait perspective

The trait perspective suggests that personality is determined genetically. Characteristics are likely to be shown in all situations so behaviour can be predicted. Trait psychologists suggest that personality is stable and enduring. This approach does not consider that environmental learning may have an effect on the performer, or that people may consciously structure their own personalities. This illustrates the **nature** (trait) **versus nurture** (social learning) **debate**.

Eysenck's model

Eysenck suggested that an individual's personality lies upon two continua: between extroversion and introversion; and between stability and neurosis.

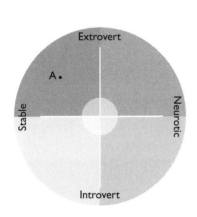

Extrovert	Introvert
• Outgoing • Likes social situations • Likes performing to an audience • Becomes bored easily as reticular activating system (RAS) is not easily stimulated	• Reserved • Dislikes social situations • Dislikes performing to an audience • Is easily over-aroused as RAS is highly stimulated
Stable	**Neurotic**
• Reliable • Consistent • Calm	• Unpredictable • Restless • Volatile

The four quadrants in Eysenck's model can be used to describe personality. For example, a stable extrovert (performer A in the diagram) is even-tempered and outgoing, while a stable introvert is consistent and reserved. A neurotic extrovert is ill-tempered and lively while a neurotic introvert is unpredictable and shy.

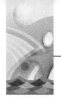

Narrow band

This theory also suggests that personality is innate and of two types.

Type A	Type B
• High stress/arousal level	• Low stress/arousal level
• Very competitive	• Not concerned with competition
• Lacks tolerance	• Very patient
• Needs to be in control of the task	• Does not need to be in control of the task
• Fast worker	• Works slowly

Social learning perspective

This approach suggests that personality is learned from experiences and changes according to the situation, so behaviour cannot be predicted. We observe and copy the behaviour and personality of significant others, such as parents, peers, coaches and role models. **Socialisation** also plays an important part (see Attitudes, below). If behaviour is successful or is praised, we are likely to imitate it. We are also more likely to copy the behaviour and personality of people who share characteristics such as gender, age and ability.

Interactionist perspective

The interactionist theory suggests that personality is determined by both traits and the influence of environmental experiences. Behaviour is a function of an individual's personality traits and the environment. A performer will adapt to the situation. For instance, a generally introverted rhythmic gymnast will display extrovert characteristics to appeal to the judges during competition.

Personality profiling

Methods that have been used to measure personality include observation, questionnaires such as the profile of mood states (POMS), and biological testing such as heart-rate monitoring. Profiling has, however, been relatively unsuccessful.

> **Tip** When evaluating the theories of personality, make sure your examples relate specifically to personality — trait, social learning and interactionist perspectives are also seen in leadership and aggression.
>
> Learn about reliability and validity in relation to personality testing, and make sure you can give relevant examples.

Attitudes

An attitude describes an individual's predisposition to believe, feel and act towards an attitude object. Attitude objects are the focus on which the attitude is directed and can include other people, places, situations and items. Attitude plays an important role in the development of an active lifestyle, particularly for young people. If they hold a positive attitude towards physical activity, it is likely that they will participate.

However, a negative attitude may lead to a sedentary lifestyle and an increased possibility of developing certain diseases. Attitudes, while usually deep rooted, are not permanent and can be changed. Teachers and coaches must generate positive attitudes to encourage and maintain participation and healthier lifestyle choices.

Origins of attitudes

Attitudes can be positive or negative. They develop through experiences and often begin to form at an early age.

Past experiences

Winning matches or titles, for example, can result in a positive attitude. The individual develops a perception of his or her own ability as high, which increases confidence and helps to build a positive attitude towards active lifestyle pastimes. A bad experience, such as losing or injury, can have the opposite effect. The performer may develop low self-confidence and a perception of his or her ability as low. This may lead to a negative attitude towards physical activity as a whole, and to learned helplessness (see p. 48).

Socialisation

This describes how individuals fit in with the **cultural norms** surrounding them. It is particularly important for school-age children. If it is the norm for your friends or family to participate regularly in sport, then you will conform, because you don't want to feel left out. However, if your peers and family do not participate and hold negative attitudes, you will adopt these attitudes to be consistent with those around you. A sedentary lifestyle may result. Religious beliefs often play a major part in the development of attitudes.

Social learning

This involves imitating the attitudes of significant others such as parents, teachers and peers. If your parents and friends have a positive attitude towards physical activity it is likely that you will copy them, especially if you are praised for doing so. Conversely, if they hold negative attitudes and abstain from participating, it is likely that you will do the same.

Media

High-profile role models in the media often display positive attitudes and, as we respect them, we are likely to adopt their attitude towards being active.

The more we are exposed to positive experiences, positive role models in the media and the positive effects of socialisation and social learning, the more likely it is that we will develop a positive attitude towards physical activity and a healthy lifestyle.

Prejudice

Prejudice is a biased judgement often based on race, gender, age, physical ability, sexual orientation or negative attitudes towards officials or the police. It is detrimental to sport and can reduce participation in certain groups. Prejudice may develop due to:
- social learning and/or socialisation
- past experience
- media hype

The components of attitudes

The **triadic model** suggests that an attitude is made up of three components:

- cognitive: beliefs/thoughts
- affective: emotions/feelings
- behavioural: actions/responses

Attitudes are inconsistent. A performer may believe that attending the gym is good for him or her and enjoy it but may not attend owing to lack of time or motivation. Beliefs don't always correspond with behaviour and therefore attitudes are poor predictors of behaviour.

Changing attitudes and prejudice

It is important to be able to change the negative attitude of someone who does not participate in physical activity or who shows prejudiced behaviour. Strategies include:

- persuasive communication particularly by significant others
- ensuring positive, successful experiences
- praising positive attitudes or non-prejudicial behaviour
- punishing prejudice, e.g. substitution or bans
- using positive role models in the media to highlight positive attitudes
- merging groups so that individuals work together across gender, age etc.
- generating cognitive dissonance

Cognitive dissonance

When poeple's attitude components all match, whether positively or negatively, they are in a state of **cognitive consonance**. Their beliefs, feelings and actions are in harmony and their attitude will remain. One way to change an attitude is to create **cognitive dissonance** by generating unease in the individual. This unease is created by changing one or more of the negative attitude components into a positive, thus causing the individual to question his or her attitude.

Attitude components can be changed through:

- education using a significant other
- ensuring a positive experience
- persuasive communication

Achievement motivation

In demanding situations performers will exhibit either **need to achieve** (NACH) or **need to avoid failure** (NAF) characteristics. This is based on their personality and situational factors. It dictates the level of competitiveness shown by the individual.

NACH performer	NAF performer
• Exhibits approach behaviour • Has high self-efficacy/self-confidence • Enjoys challenges • Will take risks	• Exhibits avoidance behaviour • Has low self-efficacy/self-confidence • Dislikes challenges • Will take the easy option

NACH performer	NAF performer
• Sticks with the task until it is complete • Regards failure as a step to success • Welcomes feedback and uses it to improve • Takes personal responsibility for the outcome • Attributes success internally • Is competitive — likes tasks with a low probability of success (i.e. challenging) and a high incentive (i.e. will be extremely proud to achieve his or her goal)	• Gives in easily, especially if failing • Does not welcome feedback • May experience learned helplessness • Attributes failure internally • Is not competitive — likes tasks with a high probability of success (i.e. easy) and a low incentive (i.e. little satisfaction in achieving his or her goal)

To generate NACH:
- ensure success by setting achievable process and performance goals
- raise confidence by giving positive reinforcement
- highlight successful role models who have comparable characteristics
- credit internal reasons (e.g. ability) for success
- blame failure on external reasons (e.g. luck)

> **Tip** Short questions may ask for the characteristics of NACH and NAF perform-
> ers. Don't make the mistake of linking extrovert personalities with NACH performers
> — there are many NACH introverts!

Attribution theory

Attribution theory tells us how individuals explain their behaviour. In a sporting context, performers use attributions to provide reasons for winning or losing.

Weiner's attribution model

Weiner suggested that four key attributions lie on two dimensions:

The **locus of causality** describes where the performer places the reason for winning or losing:
- internal — within the performer's control
- external — under the 'control' of the environment

The **stability dimension** describes how fixed the attributions are:
- stable — remain the same for a relatively long period of time, e.g. a season
- unstable — change may occur from week to week or within minutes

The locus of causality

		Internal	External
The stability dimension	Stable	Ability	Task difficulty
	Unstable	Effort	Luck

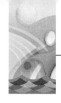

Mastery orientation

Mastery-orientated performers generally attribute success to internal reasons. Attributing in this way raises the self-efficacy of performers who will be able to repeat their success in the future. As their confidence is high, they may be motivated to continue participating. They show the characteristics of NACH performers and will persist if they do not succeed. When mastery-orientated performers fail, they attribute this to external factors such as task difficulty or luck. They then feel that failure can be overcome if they try harder.

Learned helplessness

Learned helplessness develops when performers attribute failure internally to stable reasons. They believe that, regardless of effort, they are destined to fail and therefore they do not persist. It can be general, relating to all sports, or specific, relating to one skill or to a single sport. Learned helplessness usually occurs when performers have low self-confidence due to past failings; they withdraw and stop participating. It may also be due to a coach setting unrealistic goals. Performers with learned helplessness have similar characteristics to NAF performers and if their attributions remain unchanged, they will probably lead a sedentary lifestyle because of their low sporting self-esteem.

To reduce the effects of learned helplessness, the performer should change negative attributions into positive ones. This process is called **attributional retraining**. Performers and coaches should always attribute the reasons for winning internally, to ability and effort, rather than externally, to luck, and failure should be attributed externally rather than internally. This is known as **self-serving bias**. This will raise self-efficacy and self-esteem and increase the likelihood of an individual continuing to participate.

In addition to attribution retraining, to build a mastery-orientated approach coaches should:
- set realistic process and/or performance goals
- raise self-efficacy by using Bandura's model (see p. 59)
- highlight previous quality performances
- give positive reinforcement

Aggression

Hostile aggression is when an individual purposefully harms or injures an opponent for no reason but to inflict pain.

Instrumental aggression is when an individual purposefully harms or injures an opponent but the aim is *not* to harm or injure but to gain an advantage. Anger is not involved.

Assertion is often confused with aggression. Assertion is when an individual plays hard, but within the rules, using more effort than usual. There is no intention to harm the opposition. For instance a crunching but fair tackle in rugby union is assertion.

There are many causes of aggression including:
- losing
- playing badly
- teammates not trying
- unfair officials' decisions
- provocation by an opponent or the crowd
- contact sport, e.g. ice hockey, Gaelic football

Aggression should be channelled — all the performer's effort and energy should be redirected into positive, assertive play rather than negative, aggressive reactions.

Theories of aggression

Instinct theory
As humans, we have a natural predisposition to be aggressive. Instinct theorists believe that aggression builds up within us and we require a positive outlet to release it. This is known as **catharsis**. For example, after a hard week at work you release your aggression by playing football and making several aggressive tackles. This theory has the following drawbacks:
- It does not consider the effect of environmental or social learning on aggression.
- Individuals often experience increased aggression during sporting competition rather than it having a cathartic effect.
- Some societal groups exhibit no aggression.

Frustration–aggression hypothesis

When a performer has a drive to achieve a goal but is prevented from doing so, he or she experiences frustration. Frustration always leads to an aggressive response.

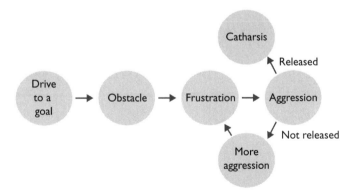

This theory does not account for:
- performers who experience frustration and aggression even when goals have not been blocked
- performers whose goals are blocked and who experience frustration but do not react aggressively

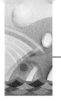

Aggressive cue hypothesis (Berkowitz)

Berkowitz updated the frustration–aggression hypothesis. When a performer has a goal blocked, his or her arousal levels increase and frustration occurs. This leads to him or her being *ready* for an aggressive act, rather than aggression being inevitable. An aggressive act will only happen if learned cues or triggers are present. For example, inherently aggressive objects such as bats or aggressive contact sports such as rugby are more likely to produce an aggressive response.

Social learning theory

This opposes the trait approach. **Bandura** suggested that aggression is learned by watching and copying the behaviour of significant others. If an aggressive act is reinforced or is successful, it is likely to be copied. Performers may also become aggressive due to socialisation. Aggression is more likely to be copied if the model shares characteristics with the performer. This theory does not, however, take into account genetic explanations as to why aggression occurs. It discounts the trait approach even though recent studies have shown that there may be an aggressive/angry gene in humans.

> **Tip** The extended question may ask you to discuss the nature versus nurture debate on aggression, or simply to describe the theories of aggression. To gain the highest marks, address the topics with clear examples.

Eliminating aggression

Performers who are repeatedly subjected to aggression may feel intimidated and stressed, lose concentration and/or self-esteem, become injured and withdraw from participating. It is therefore important that undesirable aggressive acts are eliminated from sport.

Players	Coaches
Use **cognitive** techniques • mental rehearsal/imagery/visualisation • selective attention • negative-thought stopping • positive self-talk Use **somatic** techniques • relaxation techniques • deep breathing • biofeedback General techniques • count to 10 • walk away • mantra • displace aggressive feelings by playing hard, e.g. kicking the ball harder	Praise non-aggressive acts Highlight non-aggressive role models Punish aggression e.g. substitution/fines Use peer pressure to remind one another that aggression is unacceptable Set process and performance goals rather than product goals Ensure their own behaviour is not aggressive Give the performer responsibility within the team

> **Tip** When asked for strategies to reduce aggression, give a range of answers as some will appear at the same point on the mark scheme and you will only receive credit once.

What the examiner will expect you to be able to do

- Describe the three theories of personality: trait (including Eysenck's model and narrow band theory), social learning and interactionist. Evaluate these theories and personality profiling using correct technical terminology and examples.
- Explain the three components of an attitude or prejudice and how they are formed, giving clear examples.
- Describe cognitive dissonance and persuasive communication, with examples.
- Give characteristics of NACH and NAF performers and support your answers with examples. Note the links with attribution theory and self-confidence.
- Understand and apply Weiner's model to sporting situations, define the key terms and understand the links with achievement motivation.
- Explain how a coach can reduce learned helplessness and promote mastery orientation in performers.
- Give clear definitions and examples of aggression.

Group dynamics of performance and audience

Groups and teams

A group is three or more people who:
- interact with each other, i.e. communicate
- share a common goal
- have mutual awareness, i.e. influence and depend on each other

Steiner's model of group performance

actual productivity = potential productivity – losses due to faulty processes

Actual productivity is a team's level of achievement on a specific task, for instance a netball team reaching the semi-final of a cup competition.

Potential productivity is the best possible level of achievement when the team is cohesive, for instance the netball team winning the cup competition.

Losses due to faulty processes are the coordination and motivation problems the team faces, which reduce the level of cohesion and therefore lower the level of achievement. For instance, if some team members' motivation levels are lower than expected, the team will not win the cup final.

Steiner suggested that problems affecting a team's productivity include:
- coordination problems (e.g. team members fail to communicate properly resulting in poor timing or set plays breaking down)
- lack of understanding of members' roles in the team
- lack of understanding of tactics or strategies set by the coach

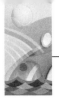

- the **Ringelmann effect**
- motivation losses (e.g. team members withdrawing effort)
- **social loafing**

The Ringelmann effect and social loafing are faulty processes that have a detrimental effect on the cohesiveness and attainment of a team. Long-term effects include performers withdrawing from and/or avoiding sporting activity altogether, leading to a sedentary lifestyle and detrimental health effects.

> **Tip** Short questions may ask you to describe a group or various aspects of Steiner's model. Learn these as they offer easy marks to pick up in the exam. Make sure that you can describe the Ringelmann effect and social loafing and give examples of both.

Group cohesion

A cohesive team has unity, a structure and everyone pulls together to reach the shared aim. The more cohesive a team is the more successful it will be, and the more successful the team is the more cohesive it becomes. There are two types of cohesiveness and the most effective groups show *both*.

Task cohesion means group members work together to meet a common aim. They may not socialise away from the team and may not share views. To achieve their potential in the sporting arena, however, they come together and can get good results. This is important in interactive sports such as football and volleyball where the team members must cooperate and rely on one another's timing and coordination.

Social cohesion occurs when group members get along and feel attached to others. They communicate and support each other inside and outside the sporting arena. This is important in co-active sports where you perform individually but your effort contributes to a whole team performance, for instance the Davis Cup in tennis.

Both task and social cohesion are reasons for being attracted to a group — other members may share your goal of winning, but you want to join because your friends are members. Or you integrate to work effectively with others towards your goal and attempt to get along socially with the other group members.

Other factors that affect the formation and development of a cohesive group include:

- Leadership style — weak leadership often results in breakdowns within a team.
- Level of satisfaction — the greater members' satisfaction with the group, the stronger the cohesion.
- Past and future success — if you have succeeded against an opponent before, you can expect to succeed again. Success increases cohesion.
- Shared group characteristics — if you are the same gender, similar age and ability, cohesion is more likely.
- Group stability — an ever-changing group is disruptive and reduces the chance of cohesion developing.

By raising cohesiveness and countering faulty processes such as social loafing, the coach can improve individual and whole-team performance. The more an individual feels valued by and part of a team, the more likely he or she is to continue to participate and therefore lead a healthy lifestyle. Coaches can:

- highlight individual performances
- give specific roles and responsibility within the team
- develop social cohesion with team-building exercises, tours etc.
- praise or reward cohesive behaviour
- raise individuals' confidence
- encourage the group identity, e.g. have a set kit
- provide effective leadership that matches the preferred style of the group
- select players who work well together rather than isolating 'stars'
- set achievable process and performance goals
- continually emphasise the team goal
- select players who are less liable to social loafing
- punish social loafing
- groove set plays to improve coordination

Leadership

Effective leaders are often ambitious, have a clear vision or goal and have the ability to motivate others to achieve that goal. Leaders may be:

- charismatic
- good communicators
- confident
- knowledgeable and/or skilful in the sport
- empathetic

Prescribed leaders are chosen from outside the group, for instance national governing bodies appoint national team managers. They often bring new ideas but can cause disagreements if group members are opposed to the appointment.

Emergent leaders are selected from within the group, often being nominated by the other group members. This person probably already commands respect, but he or she may not bring new strategies.

Leadership styles

Autocratic/ task-orientated	Democratic/ social-orientated	Laissez-faire
Dictatorial in style Primary concern is task completion Sole decision-maker Use in dangerous situations Use with large groups Use if time is limited Use with hostile groups Use with cognitive performers Preferred by male performers	Primary concern is developing relationships Group members are involved in making decisions Use with small groups Use if lots of time available Use with friendly groups Use with advanced performers Preferred by female performers	Leader is a 'figurehead' rather than an active leader Group members make all the decisions Useful if a problem-solving approach is required Only effective with advanced performers

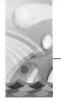

Leadership theories

The trait approach: the 'great man' theory

This approach suggests that some people are born with the characteristics necessary to become good leaders. The characteristics are innate, are shown by men rather than women, and are stable and enduring, so will be evident in all situations. There is little support for this theory as it is rare to find someone who can lead effectively inside and outside the sporting arena. The theory also disregards the effects of the environment and the fact that individuals may learn leadership qualities.

Social learning theory

This approach opposes the trait theory, leading to the 'nature versus nurture' debate. Social learning theory suggests that individuals learn leadership skills through experience by observing and imitating successful leaders.

Interactionist approach

This is the most widely accepted approach as it combines the trait and social learning theories. It suggests that leaders are born with leadership traits but they also learn and develop other characteristics through experience.

Chelladurai's multi-dimensional model of leadership suggests that leaders must be able to adapt. They must consider three factors:
- The situation — the strength of the opponents or the level of danger. For example, learning to trampoline is dangerous so requires an autocratic approach.
- Their own ability, personality and preferred leadership style. For example, an experienced leader might prefer to use an autocratic style.
- The group — ability levels, the relationships with one another and with the leader. For example, the group comprises cognitive performers and therefore needs to be given direct instructions about how to perform on the trampoline.

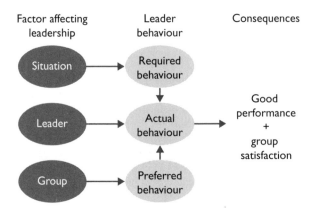

The leader must try to balance the style of leadership with each of these to gain the highest level of performance and satisfaction from the group.

Tip Many students find Chelladurai's model difficult. Try working backwards through the model, describing each box and what it means in your answer. Always give clear examples and when working through a model, use the same example throughout.

Social facilitation and inhibition

Some people enjoy performing to an audience and their performance improves. This is known as **social facilitation**. Others dislike performing to an audience and their performance worsens. This is known as **social inhibition**. These performers may lose motivation as they cannot deal with the pressure. They may avoid evaluative sporting situations and lead a sedentary lifestyle.

Tip To understand social facilitation fully you need to have knowledge of arousal. If relevant, bring arousal into your answers, particularly in extended answers.

Passive and interactive others

Zajonc suggested that four types of 'others' may be present during performance.

'Passive others' do not interact with the performer but, simply by being present, have an effect.

- An audience does not speak but watches, for instance silent observers during a tee-off in golf or a scout who arrives to observe a performance. The audience's mere presence can make performers anxious and affect their game.
- Co-actors perform the same task at the same time but do not compete against you, for instance the sight of another cyclist in front makes you speed up in order to overtake. Although you win nothing by doing so, the other's presence has made you cycle faster.

'Interactive others' communicate directly with the performer.

- Competitive co-actors are the opposition, e.g. other swimmers during a race.
- Supporters are the crowd, e.g. the spectators at a rugby match may applaud or shout abuse at performers, increasing players' motivation.

Even when passive others such as an audience are present, the main effect on the performer is increased arousal levels. The presence of an audience has the same varied effects on performance as arousal, as illustrated by the inverted U hypothesis.

Factors facilitating and inhibiting performance

Performance will be facilitated if:

- the performer is an expert and used to performing in front of an audience
- he or she is performing a gross skill
- the skill is simple and requires limited decision making
- the performer is an extrovert — extroverts have low levels of natural arousal so their reticular activating system (RAS) is activated by high levels of stimulation and they see the presence of the audience as an opportunity to 'show off' and rise to the challenge

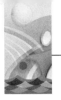

Performance will be inhibited if the performer is:

- a novice who finds performing in front of an audience intimidating
- performing a fine skill that requires precision and accuracy, which is difficult to maintain at high arousal
- performing a complex skill that demands decision-making
- an introvert who dislikes social situations and has high levels of natural arousal so his or her RAS is activated with low levels of stimulation

Zajonc based his model on Hull's drive theory, which suggests that at heightened levels of arousal, performers revert to their dominant response. This is a well-learned skill that the performers use when under intense competitive pressure.

Expert performers have motor programmes stored in their long-term memory and their dominant response is likely to be performed correctly. Therefore performance will be facilitated. Novice performers have not yet grooved their responses so the presence of an audience will inhibit their performance.

Evaluation apprehension

This is the fear of being judged. It causes the performer to revert to the dominant response. If a performer perceives that he or she is being judged, it will affect the performance. Factors that can cause evaluation apprehension include:

- a knowledgeable audience, e.g. the presence of a scout
- the presence of significant others such as parents or peers
- whether an audience is supportive or abusive, which will facilitate or inhibit performance
- naturally high trait anxiety, which will inhibit a performer in front of an audience
- low self-efficacy, which will make a performer doubt his or her ability and cause inhibition

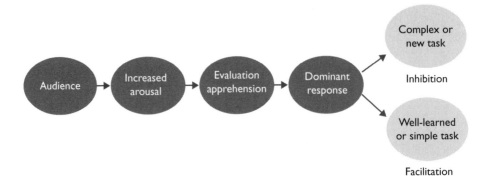

Homefield advantage

Performers usually perform better when playing at home as they have a large number of supporters, don't have to travel and are familiar with the venue. This keeps uncertainty and therefore arousal levels low. If the audience is very close to the playing area, homefield advantage is even more important, e.g. in basketball. During the later stages of a competition, however, the pressure may be high when playing at home due to the crowd's expectations of winning, therefore causing inhibition.

Baron's distraction conflict theory

This suggests that during performance we pay attention to the task in hand but we may also pay attention to 'distracters'. These could come from external sources such as the crowd or internal sources such as negative thoughts. By paying attention to both the task and the distracters, a psychological conflict is caused, which increases arousal. This leads to either social facilitation or inhibition, depending on the type of task and the performer's level of ability. For example, when taking a penalty a footballer is concentrating on the task — the ball and goal. The crowd members behind the goal cause a distraction by shouting at the player, which diverts some of his attention away from the task. This causes psychological conflict and arousal levels increase. Complex skills are likely to become inhibited as the performer cannot deal with the demands placed on his or her attention. Simple skills can be performed at a high level because the distraction can be dealt with.

Tip While it is not essential to know psychologists' names, it is desirable to give them whenever possible in the exam. It shows the examiner that you have read and understood the studies relating to this unit.

Strategies to combat social inhibition
- Familiarisation training: allow an audience to watch you training or play crowd noise during training.
- Increase self-efficacy (see Bandura's model).
- Practise skills until they are grooved.
- Selective attention: block out the crowd and concentrate on the relevant stimuli.

Use other cognitive strategies such as:
- mental rehearsal/imagery
- positive self-talk
- negative-thought stopping

What the examiner will expect you to be able to do
- Describe what a group/team is and define the various aspects of Steiner's model.
- Account for the factors relating to the formation of a group and its cohesion, including task and social cohesion, and give clear examples.
- Describe the characteristics of a good leader.
- Give clear descriptions and examples of the various leadership styles. Be able to describe all three theories of leadership and discuss the nature versus nurture debate relating to leadership.
- Demonstrate knowledge and understanding of Chelladurai's multi-dimensional model of leadership.
- Show good knowledge of arousal. Remember that the effects of an audience can be positive or negative.

The impact on performance of mental preparation

Goal setting

Psychological research has shown that setting goals has a positive effect on performance. Performers who set goals are more committed, maintain participation and are more task-persistent. The benefits of setting goals include:

- giving the performer an aim or focus
- increasing motivation when the goal is accomplished
- increasing confidence levels
- controlling arousal/anxiety levels
- focusing efforts in training and game situations

Types of goals

- Process goals are relatively short-term goals set to improve technique.
- Performance goals are intermediate goals often set against yourself to improve performance from last time.
- Product goals are long-term goals reached after extensive work. They are often set against others and are outcome based.

Short-term and intermediate goals are motivational as they are often achieved quickly. They build confidence as the performer receives feedback and therefore continues to strive towards more advanced goals. Long-term goals provide a final aim. When setting goals, it is important not to focus solely on the outcome of winning as this increases the likelihood of failure, causing anxiety for the performer and lowering motivation. Shorter term process and performance goals should be set. When running a marathon, for instance, instead of setting an unrealistic goal of winning, the athlete should aim to achieve a personal best (PB) time.

The SMARTER principles of goal setting

	Explanation	Example
Specific	The goal must be exact	Reach level 10.5 on the multi-stage fitness test
Measurable	The goal must be quantifiable	Make ten tackles in the next half
Agreed	The goal must be agreed between performer and coach	You and your coach decide to reduce your 400m time by 2s
Realistic	It must be within the performer's reach	Aim to run 10km in under 55min
Time-phased	A set period must be stated	Perform a PB time in the 100m freestyle by the end of next month

	Explanation	Example
Exciting	The goal has to be motivational	Learn to do a somersault on the trampoline by next week
Recorded	The progress has to be written down	The coach will document the height of every high jump you make

Self-confidence

Bandura's self-efficacy theory

Self-efficacy describes the amount of confidence you have in a particular sporting situation. Bandura suggested that four factors influence the level of self-efficacy shown by a performer:

- performance accomplishments
- vicarious experience
- verbal persuasion
- emotional arousal

Coaches and teachers can raise performers' self-efficacy, resulting in a more positive and successful performance. Often, individuals lead a sedentary lifestyle due to low confidence in their sporting ability. By raising their efficacy in one area, coaches may increase the performer's self-esteem and belief in their ability to master other tasks. This may lead to higher participation levels and a more active lifestyle.

For example, a young gymnast is fearful when asked to perform on a full-height beam. To increase her self-efficacy, the coach may use the four techniques described below.

Performance accomplishments	Vicarious experience	Verbal persuasion	Emotional arousal
Remind her of past success in similar situations Remind the gymnast that she performed well on the lower beam and that she didn't fall off. The width of the beam is the same so she is equally unlikely to fall	**Use a role model who shares her characteristics (ability, gender, age etc.)** Ask a gymnast of similar age and standard to perform on the beam. The young gymnast will feel 'If she can do it, so can I'	**Encourage her and tell her that she can succeed. Enhance this by using significant others** The coach and friends of the gymnast persuade her that they believe she can perform well on the beam	**Show her how to control arousal levels. This may include cognitive and somatic strategies** Psychological and physiological symptoms of over-arousal (increased heart rate, sweating etc.) can reduce her self-efficacy if she perceives she cannot achieve her goal. The coach tells her to mentally rehearse the moves on the beam before mounting so that she can focus and lower her arousal levels

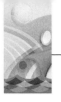

Vealey's model of sports confidence

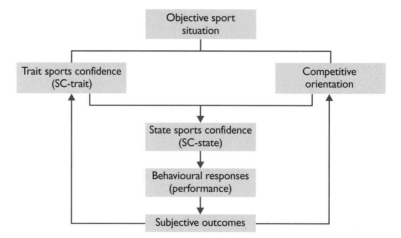

Vealey suggested that performers approach a task (the behavioural response, e.g. taking a conversion in rugby), with a certain amount of:

- trait sports confidence (SC-trait) — their natural, innate confidence level
- state sports confidence (SC-state) — their level of confidence in this situation (self-efficacy) based on past experience, e.g. a player is confident because he has kicked many conversions before
- competitive orientation — how competitive they are and the types of goals they may have set themselves, e.g. the kicker has set himself the performance goal of scoring in 90% of his attempts

The performer produces the response (e.g. attempts the conversion) and considers the subjective outcomes. If he sees the outcome as positive (e.g. a successful conversion), then the levels of general SC-trait and specific SC-state will increase. This will enhance the chances of approach behaviour being shown in other situations. A successful attempt will also increase the level of competitive orientation shown by the performer, for example the kicker's motivation grows and he sets himself a new goal of 95% success rate. A negative outcome will lower trait and state confidence along with competitiveness and may lead to future avoidance behaviour and an inactive lifestyle.

> **Tip** If you find Vealey's model difficult to understand, stick to the example of a penalty and work your way through the boxes describing both positive and negative effects.

Attentional control

During performance athletes concentrate on a range of environmental cues. If they can quickly identify, focus on and **selectively attend** to the essential elements, their performance will improve. They will avoid distraction, so reducing the risk of information overload, and reaction time will improve. They also increase the likelihood of entering the zone of optimal functioning (see p. 63).

Easterbrook's cue utilisation hypothesis links a performer's ability to sustain focus on the correct cues in the environment with level of arousal. At low levels of arousal, the performer is not stimulated enough and takes in a large number of environmental cues. He or she is unable to distinguish the relevant cues and can become confused, reducing performance level. At high levels of arousal, the performer takes in a very small number of cues and may begin to panic. The correct cues are missed, again reducing performance level. At moderate levels of arousal, the performer is able to filter out the irrelevant cues and focus only on the relevant cues. The performer completes the task to the highest level. Easterbrook therefore supports the inverted U theory of arousal, which also suggests that performance is highest at moderate levels of arousal.

Nideffer suggested that different sporting activities require different types of attentional control. For example, invasion games often require a broad attentional focus, whereas net or wall games may need a narrower style. Performers are required to apply a variety of styles, and the best athletes are able to switch from one to another readily. There are two **dimensions of focus**:
- Broad–narrow — the number of cues being focused on: 'broad' is many; 'narrow' is one or two.
- Internal–external — the location of the focus: 'internal' focuses on the thoughts and feelings of the performer; 'external' deals with environmental cues.

Four **attentional styles** arise from this:
- Broad-internal — the focus is on many cues concerning the performer, e.g. a footballer planning team strategies or the next set piece.
- Narrow-internal — the focus is on one or two cues concerning the performer; often used to calm nerves, e.g. a swimmer mentally rehearsing the starter signal and subsequent dive into the pool.
- Broad-external — the focus is on many cues in the environment, e.g. a centre player in netball focusing on several team mates prior to a pass.
- Narrow-external — the focus is on one or two cues in the environment, e.g. a basketballer focusing on the net during a free throw.

Tip Be aware of the links between goal setting, attentional control, concentration and personality.

Emotional control

Arousal describes the level of physiological (somatic) and psychological (cognitive) readiness to perform.

Arousal and performance
The inverted U theory suggests that moderate arousal levels produce optimum performance. Some performers, however, cannot tolerate much arousal while others

only reach their best performance with high levels of arousal. Similarly some skills can be performed better at low levels of arousal. This is illustrated in the diagram below.

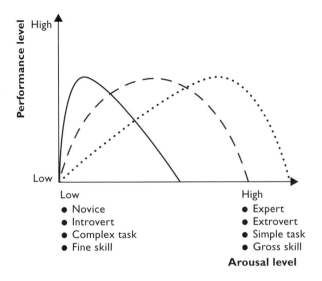

Ability level

Cognitive performers reach optimum performance at low arousal levels. They must focus on the task in hand and find competitive pressure difficult to deal with.

Associative performers can deal with moderate levels of arousal as they become more experienced. The quality of their performance increases.

Autonomous performers can deal with, and often require, high levels of arousal to reach optimum performance because they are experienced in dealing with competition effects such as the crowd's presence.

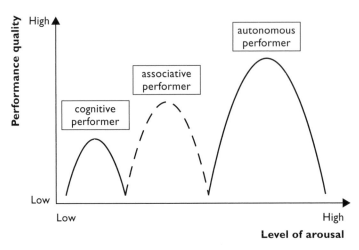

Peak flow experience

Peak flow describes the positive psychological state of performers when:

- the challenge matches their skill level
- they have a clear goal
- they have the correct attentional style
- they have a positive attitude
- they have control of their arousal levels

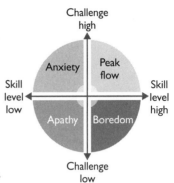

Hanin's zone of optimal functioning (ZOF)

The **zone** is a mental state that autonomous performers experience when everything is 'perfect'. Characteristics of the zone include:

- performing at optimum arousal levels
- feeling completely calm
- complete attentional control — fully concentrated on the task with the correct attentional style
- performing on 'autopilot'
- confident that success is inevitable
- performing smoothly and efficiently

Hanin suggests that optimum performance is reached during a band or zone, not at a point as described by inverted U theory. A cognitive performer or someone performing a fine skill such as a darts throw enters the zone at low levels of arousal. An associative performer or someone performing a skill that requires a certain level of precision such as a tennis serve is in the zone at moderate levels of arousal. Autonomous performers used to performing in competitive circumstances enter the zone at high levels of arousal. Gross skills such as a rugby tackle also need high levels of arousal and would be in this band.

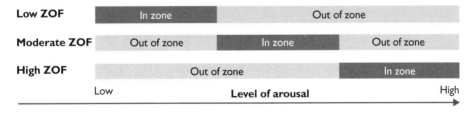

Anxiety

Anxiety affects performance negatively. It is caused by a performer's *perception* that he or she has insufficient ability. The performer begins to worry, loses focus and experiences negative thoughts that affect performance.

- Trait anxiety is where the performer is naturally anxious in all situations. It is innate, stable and enduring.
- State anxiety is where the performer is anxious only in certain situations, often caused by negative past experiences. It is a temporary feeling but it is equally

detrimental to performance. It is often seen in high-pressure situations such as taking a penalty.

The causes of anxiety include:
- task importance, e.g. playing in a final
- losing or fear of failing
- perceived inaccuracy of an official's decisions
- being fouled
- injury or fear of being injured
- lack of self-confidence or self-efficacy
- audience effects, e.g. an abusive crowd
- evaluation apprehension (see p. 56)

There are two types of anxiety
- Cognitive anxiety is the mental aspect of anxiety, e.g. worrying, irrational thoughts and confusion. Learned helplessness may occur (see p. 48).
- Somatic anxiety is the physiological aspect of anxiety, e.g. increased heart rate, blood pressure, sweat levels and muscle tension.

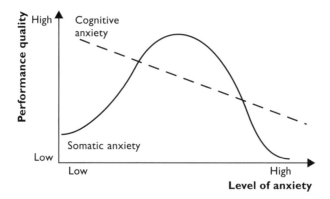

Cognitive and somatic anxiety often occur together in sport. To achieve the best performance, athletes need low levels of cognitive anxiety. They should not be worried about performing. As described in the inverted U theory, moderate levels of somatic anxiety produce the best performance.

Managing anxiety
Many performers experience high levels of anxiety when participating. If they fail to manage their anxiety, they may well stop participating. Performers can learn a range of strategies to manage anxiety levels.

Strategies for managing cognitive anxiety include:
- mental rehearsal
- imagery
- positive self-talk
- negative-thought stopping

- rational or positive thinking
- selective attention

Strategies for managing somatic anxiety include:
- progressive muscular relaxation
- breathing techniques
- biofeedback

> **Tip** Make sure you understand the strategies for managing anxiety and learn some sporting examples that you can use in the exam.

Coaches' strategies include:
- set SMARTER performance and process goals, not product goals (see p. 58)
- ensure success by setting easy targets
- ensure skills are over-learned
- raise self-efficacy (see p. 59)
- give positive reinforcement
- remind the performer of successful past experiences
- encourage performers to attribute success internally

What the examiner will expect you to be able to do

- Describe the types of goals and the SMARTER principle and give examples of all types of goal. Understand that process/performance goals are as important as 'to win' goals.
- Understand that goal setting is important in mental preparation and for developing confidence, concentration and emotional control. Be able to refer to goal setting in answers on these subjects and others such as achievement motivation.
- Understand the four key components of Bandura's model and give clear examples. Understand the key components of Vealey's model.
- Describe and apply clear examples to Easterbrook's and Nideffer's models. Be aware of the links with arousal, emotional control and selective attention.
- Show understanding of arousal and distinguish between cognitive and somatic anxiety, the causes of them and how to eliminate them.
- Understand and be able to explain the difference between state and trait anxiety.

Option B2: Biomechanics

Linear motion

Linear motion is motion in a straight or curved line. All body parts move the same distance at the same speed in the same direction.

Mechanical concepts in linear motion

Newton's laws of motion

Newton's first law of motion:

A body continues in its state of rest or motion in a straight line, unless compelled to change that state by external forces exerted upon it.

Newton's second law of motion:

The rate of change of momentum of a body (or the acceleration for a body of constant mass) is proportional to the force causing it and the change that takes place in the direction in which the force acts.

Newton's third law of motion:

To every action there is an equal and opposite reaction.

Measurements used in linear motion

- Mass is a physical quantity expressing the amount of matter in a body. Our mass is made up of bone, muscle, fat, tissue and fluid and is measured in kilograms.
- Weight is the force on a given mass due to gravity.
- Inertia is the resistance an object has to a change in its state of motion.
- Distance is the length of the path a body follows when moving from one position to another.
- Displacement is the length of a straight line joining the start and finish points.
- Speed is the rate of change of position. It can be calculated as follows:

$$\text{speed (m s}^{-1}) = \frac{\text{distance covered (m)}}{\text{time taken (s)}}$$

- Velocity is the rate of change of displacement. This means it is a more precise description of motion and is a vector quantity. It can be calculated as follows:

$$\text{velocity (m s}^{-1}) = \frac{\text{displacement (m)}}{\text{time taken (s)}}$$

- Acceleration and deceleration refer to a rate of change of velocity.
- Momentum is the product of the mass and velocity of an object.

These measurements can be split into two groups:
- Scalar quantities are described in terms of size or magnitude — e.g. mass, inertia, distance and speed.
- Vector quantities are described in terms of size and direction — e.g. weight, acceleration, deceleration, displacement, velocity and momentum.

Graphs of motion

For your exam you need to be able to plot, interpret and make calculations from three types of graph — distance/time, speed/time and velocity/time graphs.

Distance/time graphs

This type of graph shows the distance travelled over a period of time.

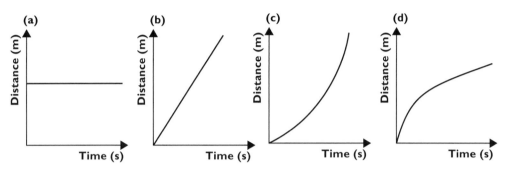

- In graph (a) the line is horizontal. This means the body must be stationary. It could represent a netball player taking a shot or a goalkeeper in football before a penalty is taken.
- In graph (b) the line goes up in a constant diagonal direction. This indicates that the performer is running the same distance over the same amount of time so his or her speed must be constant. This could occur in the middle of a long-distance race.
- In graph (c) the line is curved and gradually gets steeper. This indicates that more distance is being covered in a certain amount of time so the performer must be accelerating, for example at the start of a race.
- In graph (d) the curve starts to level off and less distance is travelled in a certain amount of time. This means deceleration is occurring, which would happen once the performer has crossed the finishing line.

Gradients of graphs

The **gradient** of a graph (its slope) is determined by:

$$\frac{\text{changes in the } y\text{-axis}}{\text{changes in the } x\text{-axis}}$$

For example, in the above graphs:
- (a) — there is no gradient, so there is no movement
- (b) — the gradient is constant, so speed is constant
- (c) — the gradient is increasing, so speed is increasing
- (d) — the gradient is decreasing, so speed is decreasing

Velocity/time graphs and speed/time graphs

These graphs indicate the velocity or speed of a performer or object per unit of time. The gradient of the graph will help you to decide whether the performer is travelling at a constant velocity, accelerating or decelerating.

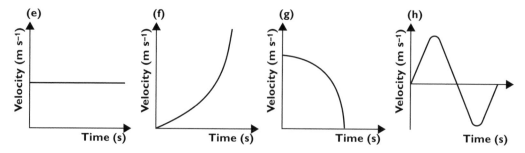

- In graph (e) the gradient is zero, which indicates that the performer is travelling at a constant velocity.
- In graph (f) the gradient gets steeper (increases). This indicates that the performer is moving with increasing velocity, or accelerating.

$$\text{gradient of graph} = \frac{\text{change in velocity}}{\text{time}}$$

- In graph (g) the gradient decreases. This shows the performer is moving with decreasing velocity, or decelerating.
- In graph (h) the curve appears below the *x*-axis. This means there has been a change in direction.

What the examiner will expect you to be able to do

- Understand Newton's laws and apply them to sporting examples.
- Understand linear motion through definitions, equations, calculations and units of measurement for mass, distance, displacement, speed, velocity and acceleration.
- Plot and interpret graphs of motion and calculate gradients.

Force

Forces and vectors

Force is a vector quantity. Remember, a vector has size and direction. Both vertical and horizontal forces act upon a sports performer.

Vertical forces
- Weight (W) is a gravitational force that the Earth exerts on a body, pulling it towards the centre of the Earth or effectively downwards.
- Reaction (R) occurs whenever two bodies are in contact with each other.

Horizontal forces
- Friction (F) occurs when two bodies in contact with each other have a tendency to slip or slide over each other. Friction acts in opposition to motion.
- Air resistance (AR) opposes the motion of a body travelling through the air. It depends on the velocity, cross-section, shape and surface characteristics of the

moving body. Air resistance is sometimes referred to as 'drag'. The degree of drag depends on the factors above and on the type of fluid environment through which the body is travelling. Compare running in water to running on land: there is a much greater drag force in water due to its greater density.

How forces act upon the body: free body diagrams

For the exam you need to know how forces are applied in sporting activities. Using free body diagrams, you can show the forces acting on a body in the form of an arrow. The length of the arrow reflects the size of the force.

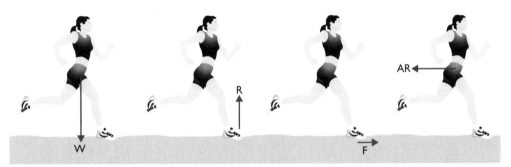

Net force is the resultant force acting on a body. Net force is often discussed in terms of balanced versus unbalanced forces.

A **balanced force** is when two or more forces acting on a body are equal in size but opposite in direction. In this case there is zero net force, and therefore no change in the state of motion.

An **unbalanced force** is when a force acting in one direction on a body is larger than a force acting in the opposite direction.

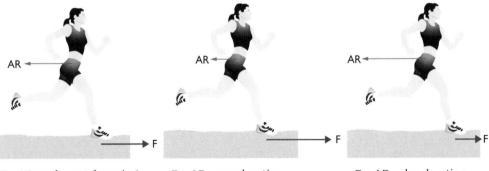

$F = AR$ so the net force is 0 $F > AR$ = acceleration $F < AR$ = deceleration

Impulse

Impulse is the product of the average magnitude of a force acting on a body and the time for which that force acts. It is equivalent to the change in momentum. In a sporting environment impulse can be used to add speed to a body or object, or to slow it down on impact. Impulse can be calculated as follows:

impulse (newton seconds/Ns) = force × time

Impulse is represented by a force/time graph. The graphs below show various stages of a 100 m sprint. It is important to note that in running/sprinting, positive impulse occurs for acceleration at take-off, whereas negative impulse occurs when the foot lands to provide a braking action.

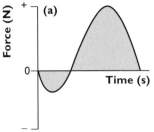

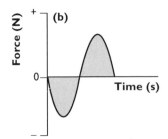

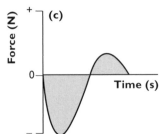

Start of the race
The net impulse is positive, which shows the sprinter is accelerating.

Middle of the race
Positive and negative impulses are equal (net impulse zero). This means there is no acceleration or deceleration, so the sprinter is running at constant velocity.

End of the race
The net impulse is negative, which shows that the sprinter is decelerating.

What the examiner will expect you to be able to do

- Give definitions and measurements of force and identify the effects of a force.
- Understand the types of force — weight, reaction, friction and air resistance — and apply these to running, jumping, throwing, hitting and kicking.
- Know how to sketch free body diagrams showing all the vertical and horizontal forces acting on a performer.
- Understand net forces through definitions and application of balanced and unbalanced forces.
- Understand impulse and the relationship it has with increasing and decreasing momentum.
- Represent impulse on a graph.

Projectiles

Projectile motion is the motion of an object, or the human body, as it is projected into the air at an angle. Three factors determine the horizontal distance that a projectile will travel:

- angle of release
- velocity of release
- height of release

Forces affecting projectiles

Weight and air resistance are the two forces that affect projectiles while they are in the air. Projectiles with a large weight have a small air resistance and follow a parabolic flight path.

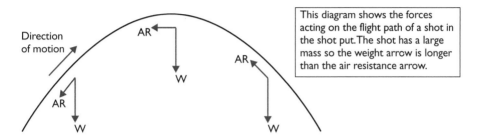

This diagram shows the forces acting on the flight path of a shot in the shot put. The shot has a large mass so the weight arrow is longer than the air resistance arrow.

Projectiles with a lighter mass, such as a shuttlecock, are affected by air resistance much more and this causes them to deviate from the parabolic pathway.

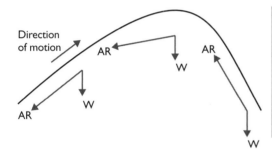

This diagram shows the forces acting on the flight path of a shuttlecock. Compared with the shot, the shuttlecock has a lighter mass and an unusual shape, which increases its air resistance. In a serve the shuttlecock starts off with a high velocity provided by the force of the racket. As the shuttlecock continues its flight path, it slows down and the effect of air resistance decreases.

Parallelogram of forces

We now know that weight and air resistance are the two forces acting on a projectile. The effect of these two forces can be represented by a single resultant force. To work out the size and direction of this resultant force, a parallelogram of forces is used. This is shown below; the diagram depicts the start of the flight path of a shot in the shot put.

To work out the resultant force:
- Draw the two force arrows of weight and air resistance, giving them direction. Remember to consider the mass, velocity and cross-sectional area of the projectile as this will determine the length of your arrows.
- Draw in the missing sides of the parallelogram geometrically (dotted lines).
- Draw a diagonal arrow from the origin of the forces to the opposite corner of the parallelogram (dashed arrow). This is the resultant force and is in a similar

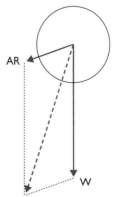

direction to the weight arrow of the shot. This means that air resistance is negligible and the shot will follow a flight path close to a true parabola.

With a table-tennis ball the weight arrow would be shorter than that for the shot, because a table-tennis ball is lighter. There will be more air resistance, so this arrow is longer. Now the resultant force is in a similar direction to air resistance, which will result in the table-tennis ball deviating from a true parabola. This is highlighted in the diagram below:

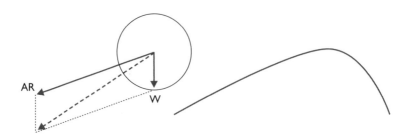

Projectiles and lift

The more lift a projectile has during flight, the longer it will stay in the air and the further it will travel horizontally. Lift is achieved when different air pressures act on an object. Air that travels faster has a lower pressure than air that travels slower. This is the **Bernoulli principle**. If this is applied to the discus, the point of release should be at an angle where the air that travels over the top of the discus has to travel a longer distance than the air underneath. This results in the air above the discus travelling at a faster velocity, which creates a lower pressure. This lower pressure above the discus creates an upward lift force and allows the discus to stay in the air for longer, resulting in a greater horizontal distance.

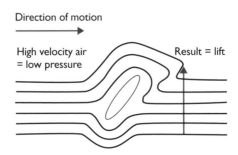

The Bernoulli principle can also be used to describe a downward lift force, such as that required by speed skiers, cyclists and racing cars. The car, bike and skis need to be pushed down into the ground so a greater frictional force is created. In a racing car, for example, the spoiler is angled so the lift force can act in a downward direction.

Projectiles and spin

Spin is imparted onto a projectile by applying a force outside the centre of mass of an object (i.e. eccentric force). For your exam you need to be aware of three types of spin.

Top spin

In tennis, for example, top spin is created when a force is applied over the top of the centre of mass of a ball. It causes the ball to rotate forwards, resulting in it dipping and a reduction in the distance travelled. When the ball hits the ground, however, it bounces forward quickly at a low angle from the ground. This increase in speed is used to try to beat the opponent.

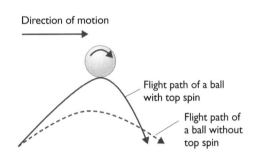

Back spin

Back spin is created in golf when the force is applied underneath the centre of mass. It causes the golf ball to rotate backwards resulting in it floating and travelling further in the air. When the ball lands, it bounces up at a large angle from the ground, its speed decreases and it stops quickly or travels backwards. This allows the golfer to have control over the landing of the ball. Back spin is also used in tennis for the drop shot.

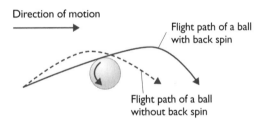

Side spin

Whether a ball goes to the left or the right depends on the position of application of the eccentric force. The diagrams below show the top view of side spin:

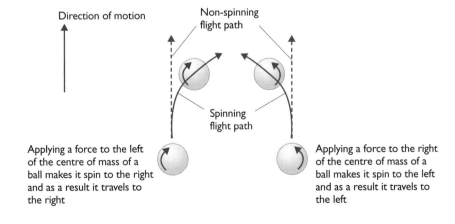

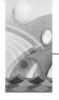

The Magnus effect

The Magnus effect is concerned with the deviation of the flight path of a spinning projectile towards the direction of the spin. It is crucial in many sports: in golf it is important to control the landing of a ball, in tennis it is used to outwit an opponent and in football it is used to bend a free kick around the wall of defenders. The Magnus effect can affect the flight path of a spinning ball as described below.

When top spin is applied to a ball, the surface at the top of the ball is travelling in the opposite direction to airflow. This means the air slows down and a high pressure is created. At the bottom of the ball, the surface is travelling in the same direction as the airflow so the air accelerates and a lower pressure is created (Bernoulli effect). This difference in pressure causes the ball to move towards the area of low pressure (bottom surface). This means the ball dips and the distance travelled decreases.

With back spin the surface at the top of the ball is travelling in the same direction as airflow. This means the air accelerates and the pressure drops. The surface at the bottom of the ball now travels in the opposite direction to airflow, so the air slows down and pressure increases (Bernoulli effect). This means that the ball moves to the area of low pressure at the top of the ball, which results in the ball floating and the distance travelled increasing.

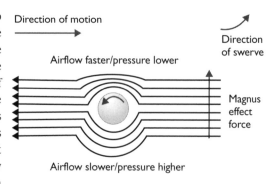

Direction of motion

Direction of swerve

Airflow faster/pressure lower

Magnus effect force

Airflow slower/pressure higher

What the examiner will expect you to be able to do

- Understand parabolas, flight paths and the forces acting during flight.
- Know how to resolve the forces acting during flight using a parallelogram of forces to explain variations in flight path.
- Describe, explain and apply the Bernoulli principle.
- Understand the types of spin in sport (top, back and side), and how spin is imparted to projectiles.
- Give an explanation of the Magnus effect and how it causes deviations in flight.

Stability and angular motion

Centre of mass

The centre of mass is the point of concentration of mass, or the point of balance. In the human body the centre of mass cannot be defined easily due to its irregular shape and as the body moves the centre of mass changes. The centre of mass for someone in a standing position is in the hip region. Males have more weight concentrated in the shoulders and upper body so their centre of mass is slightly higher than in females, who have more body weight concentrated at the hips.

A balanced stable position depends on:
- the centre of mass being over the base of support
- the line of gravity running through the middle of the base of support
- the number of contact points — the more there are, the more stable the person is; for instance a headstand has more contact points than a handstand, so is a more balanced position
- the mass of the performer — the greater the mass, the more stability there is

If you lower your centre of mass your stability increases, but if your centre of mass moves near to the edge of the base of support, you start to overbalance. A sprinter in the 'set' position will have her centre of mass right at the edge of the area of support. As she moves on hearing the starting pistol, she lifts her hands off the ground and becomes off-balanced. This allows her to fall forward and creates the speed required to leave the blocks speedily.

When performing the Fosbury flop in the high jump, the performer's centre of mass passes under the bar while his body goes over. This technique is effective compared with the scissor kick, where the centre of mass remains in the body and therefore has to be lifted over the bar.

Levers

A lever consists of three main components: a pivot (fulcrum); the weight to be moved (resistance); and a source of energy (effort or force). Our skeleton forms a system of levers that allows us to move. The bones act as the levers, the joints are the fulcrums and the effort is provided by the muscle.

A lever has two main functions:
- to increase the speed at which a body can move
- to increase the resistance a given effort can move

Classification of levers
- First-order levers — the fulcrum is between the effort and the resistance. This type of lever can increase the effects of the effort and the speed of a body, for example in the elbow during extension of the arm.
- Second-order levers — the resistance lies between the fulcrum and the effort. This type of lever is generally thought to increase only the effect of the effort force. Plantarflexion of the ankle involves the use of a second-order lever.
- Third-order levers — these are responsible for the majority of movements in the human body. They can increase the body's ability to move quickly but in terms of applying force, they are very inefficient. Here the effort lies between the fulcrum and the resistance, as seen in the forearm during flexion.

Force arm — the shortest perpendicular distance between the fulcrum and the application of force (effort).

Resistance arm — the shortest perpendicular distance between the fulcrum and the resistance.

The force and resistance arms can be seen in the third-order lever below:

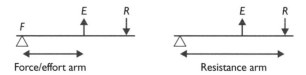

When the resistance arm is greater than the force arm, the lever system is at a **mechanical disadvantage**. This means that the lever system cannot move as heavy a load but can move the load faster. **Mechanical advantage** is when the force arm is longer than the resistance arm. This means that the lever system can move a large load over a short distance and requires little force.

Length of lever
Most levers in the body are third-order levers, where the resistance arm is always greater than the effort arm (mechanical disadvantage). The longer the resistance arm of the lever, the greater the speed at the end of it. This means that if the arm is fully extended when bowling or passing, the ball will travel with more force and therefore more speed. The use of a cricket bat, racket or golf club effectively extends the arm and allows more force.

Moment of force, or torque

Torque (or 'moment') can be described as a rotational force. It causes an object to turn about its axis of rotation. Increasing the size and the perpendicular distance of the force from the pivotal point (axis of rotation) will increase the moment of the force. Moment of a force or torque can be calculated as follows:

$$\text{moment of force or torque (newtons)} = \text{force (newtons)} \times \text{perpendicular distance from the fulcrum (metres)}$$

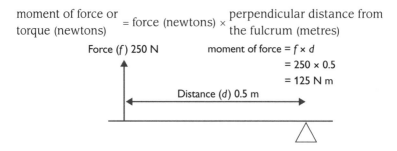

Principle of moments
When a lever system is balanced, the moment of force acting in a clockwise direction is equal to the moment of force acting in an anti-clockwise direction. The principle of

moments applies to any lever system that is balanced. An example of a balanced lever system is one that is stationary with no rotation about the fulcrum. This can be seen in the diagram below, which represents a gymnast holding a pike position on the rings:

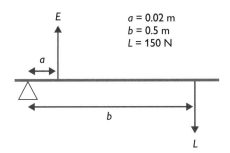

Using the principle of moments, the effort required by the hip flexors to hold the gymnast in position can be calculated:

clockwise moment of force = anti-clockwise moment of force

$$L \times b = E \times a$$
$$150 \times 0.5 = E \times 0.02$$
$$75 = E \times 0.02$$
$$75 \div 0.02 = E$$
$$3750 = E$$

So the effort required is 3750 N.

Axes of rotation

There are three axes of rotation:
- the transverse axis runs from side to side across the body, e.g. a front somersault involves rotation about the transverse axis
- the frontal axis runs from front to back, e.g. a cartwheel involves rotation about the frontal axis
- the longitudinal axis runs from top to bottom, e.g. a spinning ice skater rotates about the longitudinal axis

Angular motion

Angular motion is movement around a fixed point or axis. Angular motion occurs when a force is applied outside the centre of mass (eccentric force).

Measurements used in angular motion

Angular distance is the angle rotated about an axis when moving from one position to another. Angular distance is measured in radians (1 radian = 57.3 degrees).

Angular displacement is the smallest change in angle between the starting and finishing points, also measured in radians.

Angular speed is the time it takes to turn through an angle. It is calculated as:

$$\text{angular speed (rad s}^{-1}) = \frac{\text{angular distance (rad)}}{\text{time taken (s)}}$$

Angular velocity is a vector quantity as it makes reference to direction. It refers to the angular displacement covered in a certain time and is calculated as:

$$\text{angular velocity (rad s}^{-1}) = \frac{\text{angular displacement (rad)}}{\text{time taken (s)}}$$

Angular acceleration is the rate of change of angular velocity over time. It is calculated as:

$$\text{angular acceleration (rad s}^{-2}) = \frac{\text{change in velocity (rad s}^{-1})}{\text{time taken (s)}}$$

Newton's laws of motion related to angular motion

Newton's laws of motion can also be applied to rotating bodies by amending the terminology:

Newton's first law

A rotating body will continue in its state of angular motion unless an external force (torque) is exerted upon it.

Example: a spinning ice skater will continue to spin until she lands. The ice then exerts an external force (torque) on the skater, which changes her state of angular momentum.

Newton's second law

The rate of change of angular momentum of a body is proportional to the force (torque) causing it and the change that takes place in the direction in which the force (torque) acts.

Example: leaning forwards from a diving board will create more angular momentum than standing straight.

Newton's third law

When a force (torque) is applied by one body to another, the second body will exert an equal and opposite force (torque) on the other body.

Example: when a diver changes from a tuck to a lay-out position, he rotates his trunk back (extends the trunk). The reaction is for the lower body to rotate in the opposite direction (extension at the hips).

Moment of inertia

Moment of inertia is the resistance of a body to angular motion (rotation). It depends on the mass of the body and the distribution of mass around the axis. The closer the mass is to the axis of rotation, the easier it is to turn so the moment of inertia is low. Increasing the distance of the distribution of mass from the axis of rotation will increase the moment of inertia.

Angular momentum

Angular momentum is motion around an axis (rotation). It depends on the moment of inertia and angular velocity. These two quantities are inversely proportional: if moment of inertia increases, angular velocity decreases and vice versa.

Conservation of angular momentum

Angular momentum is a conserved quantity — it stays constant unless an external torque (force) acts upon it (Newton's first law). When a figure-skater performs a spin, turning on a longitudinal (vertical) axis, there is very little resistance to movement since ice is an almost friction-free surface. So the figure skater can manipulate his moment of inertia to increase or decrease spin speed. At the start of the spin his arms and leg are stretched out. This increases their distance from the axis of rotation, resulting in a large moment of inertia and a large angular momentum to start the spin — rotation (angular velocity) is slow.

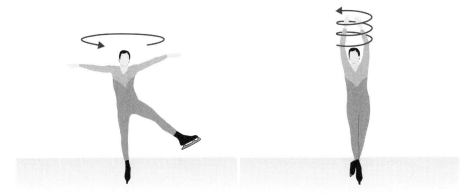

When the skater brings his arms and legs back in line with his body, the distance of his limbs to the axis of rotation decreases significantly. This reduces the moment of inertia, so angular velocity has to increase. The result is a very fast spin. There is no change in angular momentum until he uses his blades to slow the spin down.

What the examiner will expect you to be able to do

- Define centre of mass, explain how it relates to stability and rotation, and understand the relationship between centre of mass and different sporting positions.
- Define the three lever systems and give examples in the body of where these types of levers can be found. Explain the advantages and disadvantages of different types of levers.

- Define moment of force, or torque, and know how to calculate it with appropriate units of measurement.
- Understand the three axes of rotation: longitudinal, transverse and frontal.
- Define and give units of measurement for angular distance, angular displacement, angular speed, angular velocity and angular acceleration.
- Apply Newton's laws to rotating bodies.
- Define and explain moment of inertia and understand the effects of increasing or decreasing moment of inertia on efficiency and ease of movement.
- Define angular momentum, explain how it is controlled and sketch graphs to illustrate it.
- Formulate equations in relation to the law of conservation of angular momentum.

Option B3: Exercise and sport physiology

Energy

Energy concepts

Energy	• the ability to perform work • measured in joules • chemical energy — food • kinetic energy — movement • potential energy is stored
Work	• force × distance • measured in joules
Power	• work performed over a unit of time • a combination of strength and speed • measured in watts

Adenosine triphosphate (ATP)

ATP is the only usable form of energy in the body. The energy we derive from the foods that we eat has to be converted into ATP before the potential energy in them can be used. ATP consists of one molecule of adenosine and three phosphate groups:

Energy is released from ATP by breaking down the bonds that hold it together. ATPase is the enzyme that breaks down ATP into ADP + P. This type of reaction is an **exothermic reaction** because energy is released. A reaction that needs energy to work is called an **endothermic reaction**. Regenerating ATP from ADP + P is an endothermic reaction.

Sources of energy to replenish ATP

Each of the energy systems uses fuels to regenerate ATP. These fuels can be derived from chemical and food sources.

Phosphocreatine is used to regenerate ATP in the first 10 seconds of intense exercise. It is easy to break down and is stored in the muscle cells but its stores are limited.

Carbohydrates are stored as **glycogen** in the muscles and liver, and converted into glucose during exercise. During high-intensity anaerobic exercise, glycogen can be broken down without the presence of oxygen, but it is broken down much more effectively during aerobic work when oxygen is present.

Fats are stored as **triglycerides** and converted to free fatty acids when required. At rest, two-thirds of our energy requirements are met through the breakdown of fatty acids.

Protein, in the form of amino acids, provides approximately 5–10% of energy used during exercise. It tends to be used when stores of glycogen are low.

Carbohydrates and fats are the main energy providers. The intensity and duration of exercise plays a major role in determining which is used. The breakdown of fats to free fatty acids requires more oxygen than the breakdown of glycogen, so during high-intensity exercise, when oxygen is in limited supply, glycogen will be the preferred source of energy. Fats are the favoured fuel at rest and for long endurance activities.

Stores of glycogen are much smaller than stores of fat and it is important during prolonged periods of exercise not to deplete glycogen stores. Some glycogen needs to be conserved for later when the intensity could increase, for example during the last kilometre of a marathon.

Energy systems

There is a limited store of ATP in the muscle fibres, which is used up very quickly (in 2–3 seconds) and therefore needs to be replenished immediately. There are three energy systems that replenish ATP:
- the ATP-PC system
- the lactic acid system
- the aerobic system

The two key considerations when deciding the predominant energy system in use are **intensity** and **duration** of the exercise.

ATP-PC system

High-intensity activities lasting less than 10 seconds use the ATP-PC system. Phosphocreatine (PC) is present in the sarcoplasm of the muscles. Its ready availability is important for providing high power contractions, e.g. in the 100m. However, supplies only last for up to 10 seconds and PC can only be replenished when the intensity of the activity is sub-maximal.

When the enzyme creatine kinase detects high levels of ADP, it breaks down phosphocreatine to phosphate and creatine, releasing energy in an exothermic reaction.

phosphocreatine (PC) → phosphate (Pi) + creatine (C) + energy

This energy is then used to convert ADP to ATP in an endothermic reaction:

energy + ADP + Pi → ATP

This is a coupled reaction. For every molecule of PC broken down, enough energy is released to create one molecule of ATP. This system is inefficient but it has the advantage of not producing fatiguing by-products and it helps delay the onset of the lactic acid system.

Lactic acid system

High-intensity activities lasting approximately 1 minute use the lactic acid system. Once PC is depleted (at around 10 seconds) the lactic acid system takes over and regenerates ATP from the breakdown of glucose. Glucose is stored in the muscles and liver as glycogen, which has to be converted to glucose. This process is called **anaerobic glycolysis**. The glucose molecule is broken down into two molecules of pyruvic acid, which is then converted to lactic acid by the enzyme lactate dehydrogenase. The main enzyme responsible for the anaerobic breakdown of glucose is PFK (phosphofructokinase), which is activated by low levels of phosphocreatine. The energy released from the breakdown of each molecule of glucose is used to make two molecules of ATP.

Aerobic system

Low-intensity activities of longer than 1–2 minutes use the aerobic system. This system breaks down glucose into carbon dioxide and water, which, in the presence of oxygen, is much more efficient. The complete oxidation of glucose produces 38 molecules of ATP in three stages:

(1) **Glycolysis.** This process is similar to anaerobic glycolysis but in the presence of oxygen, lactic acid is not produced and the pyruvic acid is converted into acetyl-coenzyme-A (CoA). PFK is the most important regulatory enzyme for glycolysis. It is activated when there are high levels of ADP and AMP (adenosine monophosphate), and a low level of free phosphate (Pi).

(2) **Krebs cycle.** Once the pyruvic acid diffuses into the matrix of the mitochondria, forming CoA, a complex cycle of reactions occurs in the Krebs cycle. CoA combines with oxaloacetic acid, forming citric acid. The reactions result in the production of two molecules of ATP, carbon dioxide, which is breathed out, and hydrogen, which is taken to the electron transport chain.

(3) **Electron transport chain.** Hydrogen is carried to the electron transport chain by hydrogen carriers. This occurs in the cristae of the mitochondria. The hydrogen splits into hydrogen ions and electrons, and these are charged with potential energy. The hydrogen ions are oxidised to form water while the electrons provide the energy to regenerate ATP. This process creates 34 molecules of ATP.

Beta oxidation

Fats can also be used as an energy source in the aerobic system. First, fat is broken down into glycerol and free fatty acids. These fatty acids undergo **beta oxidation** whereby they are broken down in the mitochondria to generate acetyl-CoA, which is the entry molecule for the Krebs cycle. Fat metabolism then follows the same path as carbohydrate (glycogen) metabolism. More ATP can be made from one mole of fatty acids than from one mole of glycogen, which is why fatty acids are the predominant energy source in long-duration exercise.

Advantages and disadvantages of energy systems

Energy system	Advantages	Disadvantages
ATP-PC	ATP can be synthesised rapidly Phosphocreatine stores can be replenished quickly — (30 s = 50%, 3 min = 100%) No fatiguing by-products ATP-PC system can work for longer with creatine supplementation	There is a limited supply of phosphocreatine in the muscle (it lasts for only 10 s) Only one mole of ATP can be synthesised from one mole of PC PC resynthesis can take place only in the presence of oxygen (i.e. when intensity of exercise is reduced)
Lactic acid	ATP can be regenerated quickly since there are few chemical reactions In the presence of oxygen, lactic acid can be converted back into liver glycogen or used as a fuel through oxidation into carbon dioxide and water It can be used for a sprint finish (to produce an extra burst of energy)	The accumulation of lactic acid in the body denatures enzymes, preventing them from increasing the rate at which chemical reactions take place
Aerobic	More ATP can be produced There are no fatiguing by-products (only carbon dioxide and water) Glycogen and triglyceride stores are plentiful so exercise can last for a long time	This is a complicated system so cannot be used straight away. It takes time for enough oxygen to become available and to ensure glycogen and fatty acids are completely broken down Fatty acid transportation to muscles is low and requires 15% more oxygen to be broken down than glycogen

The energy continuum

This refers to the continual movement from one energy system to another depending on the intensity and duration of the exercise. The ATP-PC/lactic acid threshold is the point at which the ATP-PC energy system is exhausted and the lactic acid system takes over. The lactic acid/aerobic threshold is the point at which the lactic acid system is exhausted and the aerobic system takes over. These thresholds are highlighted in the graph below.

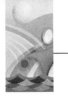

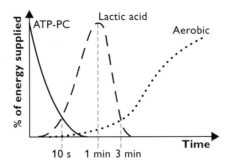

The aerobic threshold is the point at which energy can no longer be supplied aerobically and the anaerobic systems come into use.

Onset of blood lactate accumulation (OBLA)

OBLA is a good indicator of the aerobic threshold. **Lactate** is produced when hydrogen is removed from the lactic acid molecule. At rest or during aerobic exercise, approximately 1–2 millimoles per litre ($mmol\,l^{-1}$) of lactic acid can be found in the blood. However, during high-intensity exercise, levels of lactic acid rise and it starts to accumulate rapidly in the blood. When the concentration of lactic acid is around $4\,mmol\,l^{-1}$, OBLA is said to occur. Measuring OBLA gives an indication of endurance capacity. Some individuals can work at higher levels of intensity than others before OBLA occurs. OBLA is expressed as a percentage of VO_2 max. An average untrained individual will work at approximately 50–60% of VO_2 max whereas a trained endurance performer can work at around 85–90% of VO_2 max before OBLA occurs.

The multi-stage fitness test is a good practical example to illustrate OBLA. Due to the increasing intensity of this test, the performer reaches a point where energy cannot be provided aerobically. This means that the performer has to use the anaerobic systems to regenerate ATP. Blood lactate levels start to increase until muscle fatigue occurs and the performer slows down.

What the examiner will expect you to be able to do

- Define energy, work and power and identify the units they are expressed in.
- Explain the role of ATP.
- Understand the principle of coupled, endothermic and exothermic reactions.
- Explain the three energy systems: ATP-PC, lactic acid and the aerobic system. Understand the type of reaction (aerobic or anaerobic), the chemical or food fuel used, the site of the reaction, the controlling enzyme, energy yield, specific stages within each system and the by-products.
- Using duration and intensity, explain the contribution of each energy system and identify when they are used.
- Explain the energy continuum by describing how a performer interchanges between thresholds during activity.
- Explain how the following impact on the energy continuum: OBLA, availability of oxygen and food fuels, fitness level and enzyme control of energy systems.

The recovery process

During recovery the body takes in extra oxygen and transports it to the working muscles to maintain elevated rates of respiration. The surplus energy is then used to help return the body to its pre-exercise state. This is known as excess post-exercise oxygen consumption.

Excess post-exercise oxygen consumption (EPOC)

EPOC was originally referred to as **oxygen debt**. This is the amount of oxygen consumed during recovery above the amount that would have been consumed at rest during the same time.

This oxygen debt is used to compensate for the **oxygen deficit**. When we start to exercise, insufficient oxygen is distributed to the tissues for all energy production to be met aerobically, so the two anaerobic systems have to be used. The oxygen deficit is the amount of oxygen that a subject lacks during exercise.

The alactacid component (fast replenishment stage)

This involves restoration of ATP and phosphocreatine stores and the resaturation of myoglobin with oxygen. Elevated rates of respiration continue to supply oxygen to provide the energy for ATP production and phosphocreatine replenishment.

A time-out in basketball will allow for significant restoration of PC stores, thus preventing the use of the lactic acid system with its fatiguing by-product.

Myoglobin and replenishment of oxygen stores

Myoglobin stores oxygen in the muscle and transports it from the capillaries to the mitochondria for energy provision. After exercise, oxygen stores are limited. The surplus of oxygen supplied through EPOC helps replenish these stores.

The lactacid component (slow replenishment stage)

The removal of lactic acid is the slower of the two processes and full recovery may take up to an hour, depending on the intensity and duration of the exercise. Lactic acid can be removed in four ways:
- oxidation into carbon dioxide and water (65%)
- conversion into glycogen — then stored in muscles/liver (20%)
- conversion into protein (10%)
- conversion into glucose (5%)

The majority of lactic acid can be oxidised, so performing a cool-down accelerates its removal because exercise keeps the metabolic rate of muscles high and keeps capillaries dilated. This means oxygen can be flushed through, removing the accumulated lactic acid. The lactacid oxygen recovery begins as soon as lactic acid appears in the muscle cell, and continues using breathed oxygen until recovery is complete. This can take up to 5–6 litres of oxygen in the first half hour of recovery, removing up to 50% of the lactic acid.

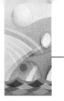

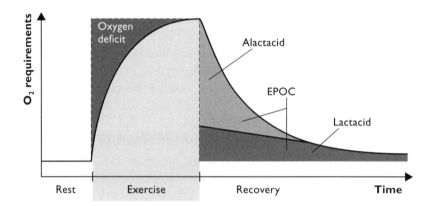

Glycogen replenishment

Glycogen, as the main fuel for the aerobic and lactic acid systems, is depleted during exercise. In addition, the stores of glycogen in relation to the stores of fat are relatively small, so it is important to conserve these in order not to cross the lactate threshold. The replacement of glycogen stores depends on the type of exercise undertaken and when and how much carbohydrate is consumed following exercise. It may take several days to complete the restoration of glycogen after a marathon, but significant amounts are restored in less than an hour after long-duration, low-intensity exercise. Eating a carbohydrate-rich meal within an hour of exercise will accelerate glycogen restoration.

Increase in breathing and heart rates

Continuing sub-maximal exercise (e.g. a cool-down) keeps hormone levels elevated. This keeps respiratory and metabolic levels high so that extra oxygen can be taken in and more carbon dioxide can be expelled from the lungs. Carbon dioxide is a by-product of aerobic respiration (see the Krebs cycle). Most of the carbon dioxide is removed in the plasma of the blood by forming carbonic acid. The high acidity is detected by chemoreceptors. These stimulate the cardiac centre and the respiratory centre in the medulla oblongata. As a result, cardiac output remains high so more carbon dioxide can be transported to the lungs and the higher breathing rate means more carbon dioxide can be expelled.

The implications of the recovery process for planning training sessions

Knowledge of the recovery process helps in planning and structuring training sessions:

- The full restoration of PC stores takes only 3 minutes, and half can be restored in 30 seconds. If athletes wish to increase their PC stores, training should not allow full recovery — for example, three sets of ten 30 m sprints at high intensity with a recovery of 30 seconds between each sprint and a recovery of 5 minutes between sets.

- Performing a cool-down decreases recovery time. Blood flow remains high, allowing oxygen to be flushed through the muscles so removing and oxidising any remaining lactic acid.
- Heart rate can be monitored to highlight when thresholds are reached. This could prevent OBLA.
- A thorough warm-up ensures that myoglobin stores are full. This will reduce the oxygen deficit at the start of exercise.

What the examiner will expect you to be able to do

- Explain EPOC/oxygen debt.
- Describe the alactacid and lactacid components of oxygen debt.
- Explain the replenishment of myoglobin and fuel stores.
- Describe how carbon dioxide is removed from the body.
- Explain the implications of the recovery process for planning training sessions.

Aerobic capacity

Aerobic capacity or VO_2 max is the maximum volume of oxygen that can be taken in and used by the muscles per minute.

VO_2 max depends on:
- how effectively an individual can inspire and expire
- how effective the transportation of oxygen is from the lungs to where it is needed
- how well that oxygen is then used

Factors affecting VO_2 max

Gender
A male endurance athlete will have a bigger VO_2 max (70 ml kg^{-1} min^{-1}) than a female endurance athlete (60 ml kg^{-1} min^{-1}). This is because the average female is smaller than the average male and females have:
- a smaller left ventricle and therefore a lower stroke volume
- a lower maximum cardiac output
- a lower blood volume resulting in lower haemoglobin levels
- lower tidal volumes and ventilatory volume

Age
As we get older our VO_2 max declines as our body systems become less efficient:
- maximum heart rate drops by around 5–7 beats per minute per decade
- peripheral resistance increases and so maximal stroke volume decreases
- blood pressure increases both at rest and during exercise
- less air is exchanged in the lungs due to a decline in vital capacity and an increase in residual air

Training

VO_2 max can be improved by 10–20% following a period of aerobic training (continuous, fartlek and aerobic interval) due to the following physiological adaptations:

- increased maximum cardiac output
- increased stroke volume/ejection fraction/cardiac hypertrophy/bradycardia
- greater heart rate range
- less oxygen is being used for heart muscles so more is available to other muscles
- maximum minute ventilation increases due to an increase in tidal volume and respiratory rate
- respiratory muscles become stronger, making breathing more efficient
- diffusion rates improve
- increased blood volume and haemoglobin/red blood cells/blood count
- increased stores of glycogen and triglycerides
- increased myoglobin (content of muscle)
- increased capillarisation (of muscle)
- increased number and size of mitochondria
- increase in the elasticity of the arterial walls, making it easier to cope with fluctuations in blood pressure
- increased concentrations of oxidative enzymes
- increased lactate tolerance
- reduced body fat
- slow twitch hypertrophy

Evaluation of aerobic capacity

The **Douglas bag** provides an accurate evaluation method under laboratory conditions. An individual runs on a treadmill to exhaustion while the expelled air is collected in a Douglas bag. The volume and concentration of oxygen in the expired air is measured and compared with the percentage of oxygen in the atmospheric air to see how much oxygen has been used during the task. This test requires access to expensive high-tech equipment.

In the **NCF multi-stage fitness test** individuals perform a 20 m progressive shuttle run in time to a beep, until they reach exhaustion. The level reached can be compared with a standard results table. This test gives only an estimate of VO_2 max and is less accurate than the Douglas bag. However, it provides a guide from which progress can be monitored, is easy to set up and requires limited equipment, making it a cheap alternative. It is also possible to test large numbers simultaneously, so it is less time-consuming than the Douglas bag.

The **Harvard step test** involves a performer stepping up and down rhythmically on a bench for 5 minutes. Recovery heart rate is recorded and used to predict VO_2 max.

The **PWC170 cycle ergometer test** involves three consecutive 4-minute workloads on a cycle ergometer. The heart rate for each workload is plotted on a graph and a line of best fit is drawn. The test is sub-maximal.

In **Cooper's 12-minute run,** an athlete runs as far as he or she can in 12 minutes. The distance covered is recorded and compared with a standardised table. In this test the performer runs to exhaustion.

Training to develop aerobic capacity

Continuous running
This is exercise without rest intervals. It concentrates on developing endurance, therefore placing stress on the aerobic energy system. Continuous training is done at a steady pace over a long period of time. The emphasis is on distance rather than speed. The duration of the run should be approximately 30–45 minutes at a training intensity of 60–75% of maximum heart rate.

Repetition running
This is used to develop speed, speed endurance and local muscular endurance. A set distance is run a specific number of times at a faster pace than continuous training and there is complete rest between runs. The speed of the repetition should be the same as if not faster than racing pace. A long-distance runner, for example, may do repeated runs of 1000 m, 1500 m, 2000 m and 3000 m to increase his or her speed.

Fartlek training
In this form of continuous training, the performer varies the pace of the run to stress both the aerobic and anaerobic energy systems. This is a much more demanding task and will improve an individual's VO$_2$ max and recovery process. A typical session will last for 40 minutes with the intensity ranging from low to high.

Interval training
This can be used for both aerobic and anaerobic training. It involves periods of work interspersed with recovery periods. It is possible to adapt interval training to overload each of the three energy systems, as shown in the table below.

Energy system	Duration or distance of work interval	Intensity of work interval	Duration of recovery	Number of work intervals/ recovery periods
ATP-PC	60 m	High intensity — 90% of max heart rate (10 s)	30 s	10
Lactic acid	200 m	High intensity — 80–90% max heart rate (35 s)	110 s	8
Aerobic	1500 m	Sub-maximal – 60–75% max heart rate (6 min)	5 min	3

Target heart rates as an intensity guide

Heart rate training zones can be used to gauge how hard you are working. Most training zones are calculated from the **maximum heart rate**. This is calculated as 220 minus your age, so if you are 17 it would be calculated as follows:

220 – 17 = 203

You then need to work at a certain percentage of this rate. One method is to use the **Karvonen principle**. This is more accurate than other methods because it takes into account individual fitness levels (resting heart rates are used to work out an individual's training zone). Karvonen suggests a training intensity of 60–75% of maximum heart rate, using the following calculation:

60% = resting heart rate + 0.6 (max heart rate – resting heart rate)
75% = resting heart rate + 0.75 (max heart rate – resting heart rate)

Energy systems and food/chemical used

It is possible to work at different levels of intensity and still use the aerobic system. The more training an individual does, the higher the level of intensity he or she can work at before using anaerobic systems. The intensity and duration of the activity will be the deciding factor in fuel usage.

Intensity of continuous running (% max heart rate)	Fuel
50–60%	Fats
60–70%	Glycogen and fat
70–80%	Glycogen

What the examiner will expect you to be able to do

- Give a definition of aerobic capacity.
- Explain how VO_2 max is affected by training, age, gender and physiological make-up.
- Describe and explain tests that can be used to evaluate aerobic capacity.
- Explain the different types of training that can be used to develop aerobic capacity.
- Identify how target heart rates can be used as an intensity guide.
- Describe which energy system and food/chemical fuels are used during aerobic activity.
- Describe the adaptations that take place after a period of aerobic training.

Strength

Maximum strength is the maximum force a muscle is capable of exerting in a single maximal voluntary contraction. It is used during weight lifting.

Elastic strength (power) is the ability to overcome resistance with a high speed of contraction. It is a combination of strength and speed.

Strength endurance is the ability of a muscle to perform repeated contractions and withstand fatigue.

Dynamic strength is the ability to apply a force repeatedly over a period of time. It is essential for explosive activities such as sprinting and is similar to elastic strength.

Static strength is the ability to apply a force where the length of the muscle does not change and there is no visible movement at a joint.

Factors affecting strength

- Fibre type. Fast-twitch fibres contract more quickly and produce more power and maximum strength. They are also designed to grow larger as a result of training.
- Cross-sectional area of the muscle. The greater the cross-sectional area, the greater the strength produced. However, two individuals with an equal cross-sectional area of muscle may produce different amounts of strength due to the lever system of the body, which in itself is determined by the position of the muscle attachment. Muscles with the largest cross-sectional area tend to be found in the legs. An individual can produce on average 4–8 kg of force per cm² of muscle cross-section.

Testing strength

Maximum strength	Hand grip dynamometer	The performer squeezes the dynamometer while lowering it from shoulder height to the side. The highest reading from three attempts is recorded
	1 rep max test	The performer lifts the maximum weight he or she can just once. It may take a bit of trial and error to find this maximum so there should be ample rest between attempts
Elastic strength (also dynamic strength)	Wingate test	The performer pedals as fast as he or she can for 30 s. The resistance on the bike is related to body weight — 75 g per kg of body weight. The number of revolutions is then recorded for every 5 s of the test
	Vertical jump	The performer's standing reach is measured against a wall. From a squatting position he or she jumps as high as possible, marking the wall at the top of the jump
Muscular endurance	NCF abdominal curl	The performer does as many sit-ups as possible, keeping in time with a beep. The test finishes when the performer can no longer keep up with the beep. The stage reached is recorded
Static strength	Isometric mid-thigh pull exercise	The performer pulls on an immovable bar (performed in a power rack with pins) as quickly as possible and maintains effort for 5 s

Training to develop strength

Improvements in strength result from working against a resistance. A strength training programme should be specific to the needs of the activity. The following factors must be considered:

- what type of strength is to be developed — maximum, elastic or strength endurance
- the muscle groups you wish to improve
- the type of muscle contraction performed in the activity — concentric, eccentric or isometric

Types of training

Weights

Weight training is usually described in terms of sets and repetitions. The number of sets and repetitions performed and the amount of weight lifted will depend on the type of strength you wish to improve. Before designing a programme it is important to determine the maximum amount of weight that the performer can lift with one repetition. Then, if maximum strength is the goal, the performer should lift high weights with low repetitions, for example, three sets of two to six repetitions at 80–100% of maximum load. If strength endurance is the goal, the individual should perform more repetitions of lighter weights, for example three sets of ten repetitions at approximately 50% of maximum load.

Circuit/interval training

Circuit training for strength can also be referred to as interval training for strength although the two methods differ slightly. Interval strength training involves completing an exercise on one muscle group then resting for 1–2 minutes before the next exercise and muscle group. In circuit training, the athlete performs a series of exercises in succession, with no rests. These exercises include press-ups and sit-up squat thrusts. The resistance used is the athlete's body weight and each exercise concentrates on a different muscle group to allow for recovery. A circuit is usually designed for general body conditioning and it is easily adapted to meet the needs of an activity.

Plyometrics

If leg power is crucial to successful performance — for example in long jump, 100 m sprint or rebounding in basketball — plyometrics improves power or elastic strength. It is based on the concept that muscles generate more force if they have previously been stretched. This occurs in plyometrics when, on landing, the muscle performs an eccentric contraction (lengthens under tension). This stimulates the muscle spindle apparatus as it detects the rapid lengthening of the muscle and then sends nerve impulses to the central nervous system (CNS). If the CNS believes the muscle is lengthening too quickly it will initiate a stretch reflex, causing a powerful concentric contraction as the performer jumps up.

To develop leg strength the performer jumps or hops over a line of benches, boxes or hurdles. Recovery occurs as the performer walks back to the start to repeat the exercise.

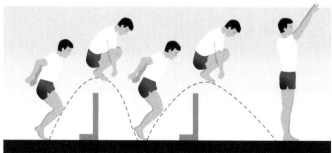

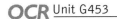

To develop arm strength, performers could do press-ups with mid-air claps or throw and catch a medicine ball.

Energy systems and food/chemical used

The table below shows the energy systems and food/chemical fuel used for each type of training.

Type of strength	Energy system	Food/chemical
Maximum	ATP-PC	Phosphocreatine
Elastic strength	ATP-PC and lactic acid system	Phosphocreatine and glycogen
Muscular endurance	Lactic acid system/aerobic system	Glycogen and fats
Static/dynamic strength	ATP-PC and lactic acid system	Phosphocreatine and glycogen

Adaptations to strength training

Neural adaptations
- More strength can be generated by the recruitment of more motor units.
- The inhibitory effect of the Golgi tendon organs is reduced, which allows the muscle to stretch further and generate more force.

Adaptations to muscle fibres
The type of strength training you do will result in specific adaptations. With weight training, for example, light weights and high repetitions allow adaptations to occur in slow oxidative fibres, whereas heavy weights and low repetitions allow adaptations in fast glycolytic fibres.

Aerobic adaptations in slow oxidative fibres include:
- Hypertrophy of slow-twitch fibres. This is where the myofibrils become thicker due to increased muscle synthesis. Hypertrophy in slow-twitch muscle fibres is not as great as in fast-twitch fibres.
- Increase in mitochondria and myoglobin.
- Increase in glycogen and triglyceride stores.
- Increase in capillaries.

Anaerobic adaptations to fast-twitch fibres include:
- Hypertrophy of fast oxidative glycolytic and fast glycolytic fibres. In addition, hyperplasia (a relatively new term) may occur whereby the splitting of muscle fibres leads to the creation of new ones. This has yet to be proven in humans but, with muscle hypertrophy, it may contribute to an increase in size.
- Increase in ATP and PC stores.
- Increase in glycogen stores.
- Greater tolerance of lactic acid.

What the examiner will expect you to be able to do

- Give definitions of the different types of strength.
- Explain the factors that affect strength.
- Describe and explain tests that can be used to evaluate strength.
- Explain the different types of training that can be used to develop strength.
- Describe which energy system and food/chemical fuels are used during strength training.
- Describe the adaptations that take place after a period of strength training.

Flexibility

There are two main types of flexibility:

- Static flexibility is the range of movement around a joint, for example doing the splits.
- Dynamic flexibility is the resistance of a joint to movement, for example kicking a football without hamstring and hip joint resistance.

Factors affecting flexibility

These include:

- elasticity of ligaments and tendons
- the amount of stretch allowed by surrounding muscles
- the type of joint — the knee is a hinge joint allowing movement in only one plane (flexion and extension); the shoulder is a ball-and-socket joint allowing movement in many planes (flexion, extension, abduction, adduction, medial and lateral rotation, and circumduction)
- the structure of a joint — the hip and shoulder are both ball-and-socket joints but the hip has a deeper joint cavity and tighter ligaments to keep it more stable but less mobile than the shoulder
- the temperature of surrounding muscle and connective tissue
- training; flexibility can decrease during periods of inactivity
- age; flexibility decreases with age
- gender; females tend to be more flexible than males due to hormonal differences

Evaluation of flexibility

The **sit-and-reach test** gives an indication of flexibility of the hamstrings and lower back. A sit-and-reach box is required. Participants sit on the floor with their feet flat against the box and legs straight, reach forward, pushing the marker with their fingertips, hold for 3 seconds and read the score. Tables are used to compare results and get a rating.

A **goniometer** can also be used to measure flexibility. This measures angles at various joints.

Flexibility training

Static stretching

- Active — the performer works on one joint, pushing it beyond its point of resistance, lengthening the muscles and connective tissue surrounding it.
- Passive — a stretch is performed with the help of an external force, such as a partner, gravity or a wall.

Ballistic stretching

This involves performing a stretch with swinging or bouncing movements to push a body part beyond its normal range of motion. This should only be performed by an individual who is extremely flexible such as a gymnast or a dancer.

Dynamic stretching

This involves controlled leg and arm swings that take a body part gently to the limit of its range of motion.

Proprioceptive neuromuscular facilitation (PNF)

First the muscle is passively stretched. It is then contracted isometrically for a period of at least 10 seconds. It then relaxes and is stretched again, usually going further the second time.

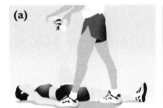
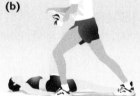
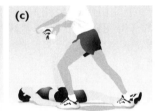

Adaptations to flexibility training

Adaptations occur after a period of flexibility training. The tendons, ligaments and muscles surrounding joints have elastic properties, which allow a change in length. There is more change to muscle tissue than to tendons or ligaments. A permanent change is known as a plastic change.

What the examiner will expect you to be able to do

- Give a definition of flexibility.
- Understand the factors that affect flexibility.
- Describe and explain tests that can be used to evaluate flexibility.
- Explain the different types of training that can be used to develop flexibility.
- Describe the adaptations that take place after a period of flexibility training.

Body composition

Body composition describes the distribution of lean body mass and body fat. On average, men have less body fat (15%) than women (25%).

Evaluation of body composition

The **skin fold test** involves taking skin fold measurements from various points on one side of the body. The measurements are added together (in millimetres) and compared with standardised tables.

In **bioelectric impedance**, a small electrical current is passed through the body. As fat offers greater resistance to the electrical current, the amount of impedance gives an estimate of the percentage of body fat.

In **hydrostatic weighing** the body is submerged in water and body mass is divided by the volume of water displaced. This calculates body density, which can be used to predict the percentage of body fat.

Body mass index (BMI) considers total body mass and is calculated as:

$$BMI = \frac{weight\ (kg)}{height\ (m) \times height\ (m)}$$

A person with a BMI of less than 19 is underweight. A BMI of more than 40 is classified as morbidly obese.

Basal metabolic rate (BMR)

This refers to the amount of energy needed by the body to sustain life while at rest. BMR decreases with age as the body's ability to burn energy slows down, but regular aerobic exercise will increase BMR. Once you are aware of your BMR, it is possible to calculate your daily calorific needs.

A rough estimation of BMR can be achieved through an equation using weight, sex, age and height. A more accurate evaluation requires gas analysis and calorimetry.

Energy balance of food (calories)

The amount of energy we need depends on the duration and type of physical activity we do. Energy is measured in calories. A calorie (cal) is the amount of heat energy required to raise the temperature of 1 g of water by 1°C. A kilocalorie (kcal) is the amount of heat required to raise the temperature of 1000 g of water by 1°C.

The basic energy requirements of an average individual are 1.3 kcal per hour for every kg of body weight. This requirement increases during exercise to 8.5 kcal per hour for each kg of body weight. Therefore, in a 1-hour training session the performer would require an extra 7.2 kcal (8.5 − 1.3 = 7.2 kcal) per kg of body weight, that is 7.2 × 1 × 60 = 432 kcal.

Diet

A balanced diet is essential for optimum performance in all sporting activities. What people eat affects health, weight and energy levels. The diet of top performers must meet the energy requirements of training and competition, as well as providing nutrients for tissue growth and repair — sports nutritionists recommend 10–15% protein, 20–25% fats and 60–75% carbohydrates.

Obesity and exercise

Obesity is defined as an excess of total body fat, usually due to energy intake exceeding energy output. Obesity increases the risk of heart disease, hypertension, high blood cholesterol, strokes and diabetes caused by a high-sugar and high-fat diet. It can also increase stress on joints and limit flexibility. It occurs when an individual's body weight is 20% or more above normal weight, or when a male accumulates 25% and a female 35% total body fat. The BMI, also a common measure of obesity, takes into account body composition. An individual is considered obese when his or her BMI is over 30.

Obese children can develop the medical problems listed above due to high-sugar/high-fat diets. They will also have weight-related issues such as lower back pain, poor posture, less mobility and flexibility, and greater stress on joints.

What the examiner will expect you to be able to do

- Give a definition of body composition.
- Describe and explain tests that can be used to evaluate body composition.
- Calculate an individual's BMI.
- Understand the term BMR and the different energy requirements of various physical activities.
- Calculate your daily calorific requirements based on your BMR and your average additional energy consumption.
- Critically evaluate your personal diet and calorie consumption.
- Understand the health implications of being overweight and how this can affect involvement in physical activity.

Application of the principles of training

Principles of training

Overload (FITT)

This is achieved by increasing one or more of the following elements.

Frequency — the number of times a performer trains per week.

Intensity — how hard a performer works. For example, the intensity of a run can be raised by increasing the pace or by running uphill. To improve aerobic fitness, training intensity should be increased above the aerobic but below the anaerobic thresholds.

One of the most recognised methods of calculating intensity is the Karvonen principle (see p. 90).

Time — the length of the session. For example, a 30-minute run could be increased to a 40-minute run. A session should last a minimum of 20 minutes.

Type — the type of training that is most suitable. For example, if the aim is to improve aerobic capacity, then continuous training would be suitable.

Progression
This involves the application of overload. It is important to overload the body in order to improve fitness but this should be done gradually.

Specificity
Training should be relevant to the sport and the individual. For example, a sprinter will do strength training on the relevant muscles and speed training to make the energy system he or she uses more efficient.

Reversibility
This is often referred to as detraining. If you stop training the adaptations that have occurred through training will deteriorate. It is suggested that aerobic adaptations are lost more quickly than strength adaptations.

Moderation
Don't overdo it. Overtraining can lead to injury.

Variance
A training programme needs to have variety in order to maintain interest and motivation.

Periodisation

Periodisation involves dividing the year into periods in which specific training occurs. These are referred to as macrocycles, mesocycles and microcycles.

Macrocycle
This involves a long-term performance goal. For a footballer it could be the length of the season or for an athlete the 4-year build-up to the Olympics. It comprises:
- the preparation period — for example, pre-season training.
- the competition period — the main aim is to optimise competition performance. Levels of fitness and conditioning should be maintained, as should the competition-specific training. In this phase, volume of training is decreased but intensity is increased
- the transition or recovery period — the athlete recharges physically and mentally and ensures an injury-free start to the season or next build-up. General, fun exercise should be carried out

Mesocycle
This describes a short-term goal within the macrocycle, which may last for 2–8 weeks. The focus could be a component of fitness. For instance, a sprinter may concentrate

on power, reaction time and speed whereas an endurance performer may prioritise strength endurance and cardio-respiratory endurance.

Microcycle

This normally describes 1 week of training that is repeated throughout the mesocycle, for instance what the performer is going to do each day from Monday to Sunday, including rest days (usually in a 3:1 ratio).

Double periodisation

Some sports require an athlete to peak more than once in a season. A long-distance athlete, for example, may want to peak in winter during the cross-country season and again in the summer on the track. A footballer may want to peak for an important club match and for an international competition later in the year. These performers have to follow a double-periodised year.

Planning a personal health and fitness programme

When planning a training programme it is important to take note of the following:
- the aim of the training programme
- macrocycles, mesocycles and microcycles
- the energy systems that need training
- the fitness components to be improved (test these first and re-test at the end to measure improvement)
- the main muscle groups used
- the type of contractions needed
- the most suitable method(s) of training
- the principles of progression, overload, specificity, moderation, variance and reversibility

What the examiner will expect you to be able to do

- Define periodisation including the macrocycle, mesocycle and microcycle.
- Plan a personal health and fitness programme that takes into account the principles of training.

Ergogenic aids

Dietary manipulation

It is possible to adapt or change your diet according to the demands of the activity.

Diet composition of endurance vs power athletes

The body's preferred fuel for any endurance sport is muscle glycogen. If muscle glycogen breakdown exceeds its replacement then glycogen stores become depleted. This results in fatigue and the inability to maintain the duration and intensity of training. In order to replenish and maintain glycogen stores, an endurance athlete

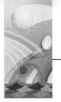

needs a diet rich in carbohydrates. Research suggests that endurance athletes need to consume at least 6–10 grams of carbohydrate per kilogram of body weight per day. Water is also essential to avoid dehydration.

In general, endurance athletes require more carbohydrates than power athletes because they exercise for longer periods and need more energy. By contrast, proteins are very important for power athletes — insufficient protein will lead to muscle breakdown. Proteins are also important for tissue growth and repair.

Pre- and post-competition meals

Before a competition

To achieve optimal performance, it is essential to be well-fuelled and well-hydrated. A pre-competition meal should be eaten 3–4 hours before competing so that the food consumed can be digested and absorbed. The meal needs to be high in carbohydrate, low in fat and moderate in fibre to aid digestion (foods high in fat, protein and fibre tend to take longer to digest). High levels of carbohydrate will keep blood glucose levels high throughout the competition.

After a competition

Most exercise will deplete stores of glycogen so it is important to replenish them. Eating a carbohydrate-rich meal within an hour of exercise will accelerate glycogen restoration.

Fluid intake

Water constitutes up to 60% of a person's body weight and is essential for good health. It carries nutrients to cells in the body and removes waste products. It also helps to control body temperature. When we start to exercise, production of water increases (water is a by-product of the aerobic system). We also lose a lot of water through sweat. The volume we lose depends on the external temperature, the intensity and duration of the exercise and the volume of water consumed before, during and after exercise. Water is important to maintain optimal performance.

Glycogen loading

This is a form of dietary manipulation involving maximising glycogen stores. Some endurance athletes use it to maximise aerobic energy production. Before an important competition a performer eats a diet high in protein and fats for 3 days and exercises at a relatively high intensity so that glycogen stores are depleted. This is followed by 3 days of a diet high in carbohydrates and some very light training. Studies show that this increases the stores of glycogen in the muscle and can prevent a performer from 'hitting the wall'.

Advantages of glycogen loading	Disadvantages of glycogen loading
Increased glycogen synthesis	Water retention, resulting in bloating
Increased glycogen stores in the muscle	Heavy legs
Delays fatigue	Affects digestion
Increased endurance capacity	Weight increase
	Irritability during the depletion phase
	Alters the training programme

Pharmaceutical aids

Creatine is a supplement used to increase the amount of phosphocreatine stored in the muscles. It is legal.
- It allows the ATP-PC system to last longer and can help improve recovery times.
- It may lead to dehydration, bloating, muscle cramps and liver damage. Studies suggest, however, that a daily intake of 5 g or over ends up in urine, not in muscle.
- It may be used by athletes in sprinting, jumping and throwing events.

HGHs are artificially produced hormones. They are illegal.
- They increase muscle mass and decrease fat.
- They may lead to heart and nerve diseases, glucose intolerance and high levels of blood fats.
- They are used across a range of sports, including sprinting, rugby and in endurance performance. The full extent of their use is unknown as they are hard to test for.

Gene doping involves synthetic genes, such as IGF-I. It is illegal.
- It can produce large amounts of naturally occurring muscle-building hormones. The use of repoxygen to increase the number of red blood cells was discovered during the 2006 Winter Olympics.
- Effects can be long-lasting and detection is difficult as the genes do not enter the bloodstream.
- It may lead to heart and liver problems.
- It is most commonly used by endurance athletes to improve oxygen uptake.

Blood doping involves removing blood from an athlete whose body then makes more red blood cells. The blood is stored and injected back into the athlete to produce a higher red blood cell count. It is illegal.
- It is used to improve aerobic capability by increasing the body's oxygen-carrying capacity, so more work can be done.
- Blood viscosity may thicken, leading to risks of clotting and death.
- It is used by endurance performers, e.g. cyclists and cross-country skiers.

Rh-EPO is a natural hormone produced by the kidneys to increase red blood cells. It can be manufactured artificially to increase haemoglobin levels. It is illegal.
- It is used to increase oxygen-carrying capacity so more work can be done.
- It can result in blood clotting and death.
- It is used by endurance performers, e.g. long-distance runners.

Cooling aids

Water

Water plays an important part in regulating body temperature. Exercise uses energy and some of that energy is released as heat. Water prevents the performer from overheating. Sweating and evaporation cool the body, but water is lost in the process. Once the body starts to lose water, there can be a drop in blood volume. When this occurs, the heart works harder to move blood through the bloodstream and the amount of oxygen available to the working muscles decreases. This will affect performance. It is therefore important when exercising to drink early and often.

Sports clothing

Manufacturers advertise clothing such as vests and caps that are designed to keep the wearer cool. The lightweight sports vest, for example, made from 'sportwool' and microfibre, is designed for body cooling. It contains a gel that can keep temperature constant for long periods. However, people are sceptical about the cooling capabilities of clothing and it is not yet widely used.

Ice baths

Ice baths are used for cooling body tissue after exercise and are a popular recovery method. Performers get into an ice bath for 5–10 minutes. The cold water causes the blood vessels to tighten and drains the blood out of the legs. On leaving the bath, the legs fill up with new blood that invigorates the muscles with oxygen to help the cells function better. The blood leaving the legs takes away with it the lactic acid that has built up during exercise. Ice baths are now used among most professional performers who train and play regularly.

Training aids

Pulleys

These are rope or small bungee-type harnesses that allow an athlete to train against a resistance. Swimmers are often attached to an elastic-type harness. They swim until the elastic is tense and try to maintain this position. If they stop or slow down the rope will drag them backwards. This method of strength training allows the exact movement pattern to be performed while resistance is applied.

Parachutes

Parachutes are used to develop speed, power and strength in the leg muscles, so developing a more powerful performance. The performer runs with a small parachute, attached to the chest by cords, billowing out behind him or her. This type of resistance training is sport-specific as it replicates the running action, thereby using the muscles in the same way.

What the examiner will expect you to be able to do

- Explain the positive and negative effects of each of the aids in this topic.
- Identify which type of performer will benefit from each type of aid.
- Explain whether the aid is legal or illegal.

Questions
&
Answers

This section of the guide contains structured questions that are similar in style to those you can expect to see in the G453 exam. The questions cover all the areas of the specification identified in the Content Guidance section. Your exam paper will have three sections and each of these will have several short structured questions, together with an extended-answer question. The extended answer will be marked by 'levels' and will include assessment of your ability to evaluate critically and to apply practical examples, the structure of your answer, and the quality of your language.

Each question here is followed by an average or poor response (Candidate A) and an A-grade response (Candidate B).

You should try to answer the questions yourself, so that you can compare your answers with the candidates' responses. In this way, you should be able to identify your strengths and weaknesses in both subject knowledge and exam technique.

Examiner's comments

All candidates' responses are followed by examiner's comments. These are preceded by the icon *e* and indicate where credit is due. In the weaker answers they also point out specific problems and common errors, so helping you to avoid pitfalls.

Question 1

Popular recreation in pre-industrial Britain

(a) One example of a popular recreation activity was mob football. Identify the characteristics of mob games. (4 marks)

(b) Modern track and field athletics have their roots in 'popular recreation' activities. Outline reasons why 'pedestrianism' was popular as a pre-industrial pastime. (3 marks)

Candidates' answers to Question 1

Candidate A

(a) Mob football was played as a popular recreation activity in pre-industrial society, which it very much reflected. There were few rules ✓ as society was illiterate. There were lots of injuries as it was a violent activity ✓ reflecting a brutal society.

> ⏀ Candidate A scores 2 marks for two characteristics of mob games. The links to features of society at the time are irrelevant.

Candidate B

(a) Key characteristics of mob games such as mob football were:
- played occasionally (e.g. on holy days) ✓
- played by males ✓
- used limited equipment naturally available ✓
- there were few rules, which were unwritten ✓

> ⏀ Candidate A scores 4 marks for the correct characteristics.

Candidate A

(b) Pedestrianism was basically race walking, which is still part of the modern Olympics today. It was a popular pastime in pre-industrial Britain because it was a simple/cheap activity to set up and organise ✓.

> ⏀ Candidate A scores 1 mark. The first sentence is true but irrelevant. There is only one point worthy of credit, linked to the idea that pedestrianism was easy to organise in a society that lacked technological development.

Candidate B

(b) Pedestrianism was popular in pre-industrial times because it was a spectacle for the public to watch as runners and walkers competed against one another ✓. The crowd liked to gamble and wager on who would win contests, which also made it popular ✓. Running and walking involved use of the land as a natural resource so it was simple and cheap to arrange ✓.

🖉 Candidate B scores 3 marks. Three correct points clearly illustrate understanding of why pedestrianism was popular in pre-industrial Britain.

■ ■ ■

Question 2

Rational recreation in post-industrial Britain

(a) **During the late nineteenth century, modern sports such as Association football replaced traditional mob games like mob football. Explain the social and economic changes that accounted for this development.** (6 marks)

(b) **Church organisations promoted sport among their local communities during the late nineteenth century. Explain their reasons for doing this and how they achieved it.** (4 marks)

Candidates' answers to Question 2

Candidate A

(a) Social factors: violence of mob games was not acceptable as society developed ✓. The Church did not like mob games and encouraged sport that had more rules and more acceptable behaviour ✓.

Economic factors: factory owners did not like mob games as they led to injury to workers ✓. If injured, workers could not work (R).

🖉 Candidate A scores 3 marks. Two relevant social factors are stated and explained to earn 2 marks. A couple more social factors would have helped ensure maximum marks on this part of the question. Only one economic factor (linked to injured workers) is made, which is repeated so can only earn a single mark. It is important to make a variety of relevant points and to avoid repetition (R).

Candidate B

(a) Socially, mob games were discouraged as they were seen to lead to gambling and drink ✓. This was frowned upon by the Church as it was against the highly moral behaviour they wanted to develop ✓. By the late nineteenth century people lived in towns and cities, which meant the traditional village rivalries of mob games had been lost ✓.

Economically, the factory system developed, which meant less time for playing sport ✓. It also meant factory owners wanted fit/healthy workers as opposed to injured ones as they lost money ✓. The damage to property mob games caused was seen as a waste of money and not acceptable in modern Britain ✓.

✍ Candidate B scores 6 marks for a well-balanced, clearly set out and structured answer that makes the necessary number of relevant points in relation to both the social and economic parts of the question.

Candidate A

(b) The Church did lots to encourage sport in local communities. They set up teams and clubs for people to play sport ✓. They also provided Church halls and playing fields on Church grounds to play sport on ✓.

✍ Candidates B scores 2 marks. This answer is too brief and only one part of the question is attempted (i.e. 'how'). Reasons *why* the Church encouraged involvement in sport should have been given to gain maximum marks.

Candidate B

(b) The Church promoted sport in their local areas for lots of reasons. These included the fact that they wanted to stop people drinking and gambling ✓. They also saw it as a good way of getting people to come to Church ✓.

To get more people involved in sport, which they now viewed in a more positive way, they organised competitions for people to take part in ✓. They also provided facilities to play in such as Church halls ✓.

✍ Candidate B scores 4 marks. Both the 'why' and the 'how' are addressed, giving this candidate the potential to score full marks. This is a relatively succinct answer but it contains the necessary detail. Being succinct is helpful in exams where effective use of time is important for success.

■ ■ ■

Question 3

The impact of public schools

(a) Public schools such as Rugby and Eton played an important part in the development of rational games in society from the mid-nineteenth century onwards. Explain the role played by the 'old boys' of such public schools in the development of rational recreation. (4 marks)

(b) Outline the reasons why the English public schools developed modern sport into its rational form from the middle of the nineteenth century onwards. (4 marks)

Candidates' answers to Question 3

Candidate A

(a) Public schools like Rugby where Thomas Arnold was headmaster were very important in the development of rational recreation as they provided specialist coaching, facilities and lots of time to play sport. They also developed muscular Christianity and athleticism to help sport develop in a rational way.

> ✎ Candidate A fails to score. This question requires a focus on the role of public school *old boys* (e.g. old boys returning as coaches), which this answer fails to mention.

Candidate B

(a) Public school old boys were important in the development of rational recreation in a number of ways. First, lots came back from university as teachers to coach games like rugby to boys at public schools ✓. Second, some became vicars and spread their love of athleticism via games in their parishes ✓. Third, as sons of factory owners, they gave facilities and set up teams to play sport to help improve the workers' health and morale ✓. Fourth, ex-public schoolboys were very important in the setting up of national governing bodies of sport that came up with rules we still play by today ✓.

> ✎ Candidate B scores 4 marks for an excellent, clearly structured answer with four clear, relevant points linked to the question.

Candidate A

(b) Sport was developed in English public schools when the original mob versions played by boys in their villages were brought to schools and then developed via a melting pot of rules into a single version played by all.

Reasons for this were that it improved behaviour both in the boys' free time at school ✓ as well as on the pitch via playing fairly ✓.

> ✎ Candidate A scores 2 marks. The first part of the answer gives correct background information on the process by which sport developed in public schools but it is irrelevant so gains no marks. The second paragraph contains two points linked to improvement in pupil behaviour on and off the field.

Candidate B

(b) Reasons why English public schools developed rational sport included the following:
- it promoted team building/loyalty in a team (e.g. via rugby football) ✓
- it developed leadership qualities in sport important to later life (e.g. captain of the rugby team) ✓
- it developed athleticism, which was a cult in public schools as it developed physical endeavour with moral integrity ✓
- it improved social control in the boys as it occupied their free time in a more positive way ✓

- it emphasised the 'taking part' as important, which encouraged sportsmanship and fair play in the boys playing games ✓

🖉 Candidate B scores 4 marks. This answer focuses on the demands of the question, identifying and briefly explaining a number of reasons why public schools developed rational sport. It makes more points than marks available to help ensure a maximum score — one may be irrelevant or a repeated point.

■ ■ ■

Question 4

Drill, physical training and physical education in state schools

(a) **How did the Model Course of military drill prepare the working classes for their role in society?** (3 marks)

(b) **The development of state PE started with the Model Course in 1902 and continued via various developments in physical training (PT) from 1904 to 1933. Identify the similarities and differences between the early state school PT syllabus developments and the current National Curriculum PE.** (6 marks)

Candidates' answers to Question 4

Candidate A

(a) The Model Course was all about getting the children to do as they were told in lessons where NCOs would shout commands at them and they would do as they were told. It was therefore important as it developed discipline important for later life ✓ as well as obedience (R) and the ability to take orders (R).

🖉 Candidates A scores 1 mark. This answer illustrates the error of focusing on a single point. This limits potential to achieve more marks. Repetition should be avoided.

Candidate B

(a) The Model Course of military drill helped to prepare children for later life in the army as many from the working class went into the army and became soldiers ✓. This required training with mock weapons to improve familiarity with them ✓. It was also important in the army as well as factories that working-class children were trained to take orders and be obedient ✓.

📝 Candidate B scores 3 marks. Three correct points are made that clearly illustrate understanding of how the Model Course helped prepare the working class for their subservient role in society.

Candidate A

(b) The Model Course was very strict and formal, taught by NCOs in classrooms. It is very different to today as we have more variety of activities taught by trained teachers in good facilities.

📝 Candidate A fails to score. The basic comparison made with National Curriculum PE is irrelevant as the Model Course preceded the PT syllabus developments asked for in the question.

Candidate B

(b) Similarities between early PT and NC PE include the following:
- both were developed and influenced by central government ✓
- both were compulsory for pupils ✓
- both had the aim of improving a child's health and fitness ✓

Differences existed between the two as NC PE had:
- lots more activities to do in lessons (i.e. more breadth) ✓
- lots more teaching styles used by specially trained teachers ✓
- lots more links to preparing children for active leisure when leaving school ✓
- lots more opportunities for pupils to use their own initiative and solve problems themselves ✓

📝 Candidate B scores 6 marks. This is an excellent answer that sets out in an examiner-friendly manner (i.e. separation of points into similarities and differences, as required by the question) a number of relevant points. It makes one more point than the maximum marks available to ensure 6 marks are gained.

■ ■ ■

Question 5

Comparative studies

(a) Explain how different historical factors have influenced the development of sports excellence in the UK compared with the USA. (4 marks)

(b) The USA has a lower rate of participation in physical activity compared with the UK. Explain why this is the case. (4 marks)

(c) Initiatives to develop and promote school **PE** and sport are important throughout the world. List and describe examples of such initiatives in the **UK** and Australia. (6 marks)

(d) The Australian Institute of Sport (**AIS**) is globally acknowledged as being a best-practice model for elite performer development. How has the **AIS** model been applied in the **UK** to develop Team **GB** athletes to fulfil their potential? (5 marks)

Candidates' answers to Question 5

Candidate A

(a) The UK has a long history of taking part in sport, with sportsmanship and fair play as strong motives for participation. This is in direct contrast to the USA where there is a Lombardian ethic with win at all costs being important in sport ✓. Britain invented most sports and we dominated them for years until other countries like America started to play them against us. This is not the case yet with football.

🖉 Candidate A scores 1 mark. Only one relevant point is made comparing the traditional ethics of participation between the UK and the USA. The other sentences are too vague or irrelevant.

Candidate B

(a) The USA has a strong spirit of frontierism and the pioneering spirit, which are reflected in aggressiveness in elite sport. This is not the case in the UK so its sport tends to be less violent in comparison with the USA, e.g. American football compared with Association football ✓.

The USA has a strong win-at-all-costs attitude that it has developed compared with the UK's early emphasis on taking part, which still exists today ✓.

In the USA, UK-invented sports have been marginalised with their own big four sports dominant to prove they are best in different sports as a new young society trying to prove itself. The UK had no such need to prove itself via sport due to its colonial past and domination of nations via the empire ✓.

The USA has historically been based on a system of merit and hard work, leading to the 'rags to riches' ideal and opportunities to rise through society via sporting achievement. In contrast, the UK has a long tradition of looking down on professionalism and paying elite performers as it was feared it would lead to negative aspects such as cheating and violence appearing in sport ✓.

🖉 Candidate B scores 4 marks for a good answer with four direct comparisons between the historical development of elite performers in the USA and the UK made in four separate paragraphs. Points are made with brief explanations that illustrate the required knowledge to achieve full marks.

Candidate A

(b) In the USA, there is low emphasis on mass participation. Few Americans get the recommended amount of physical activity in a week. This is 30 minutes pulse-raising activity five times in a week. Part of the reason for this is that the USA is more of a spectator than participator society ✓. Spectatorism dominates — watching American football and basketball on television is part of American culture, which means fewer Americans participate than in the UK (R).

> Candidate A scores 1 mark. The opening two sentences do not earn marks as they repeat the information in the question. The only relevant point (repeated again in the last sentence) links to the USA becoming a spectator society and therefore participating less.

Candidate B

(b) Americans take part in physical activity less than the British for lots of different reasons such as:
- less of an emphasis on taking part in school PE as opposed to school sport; the emphasis on winning puts some people off participating from an early age ✓
- such sporting participation is elitist with only the best feeling like they should take part and putting lots off doing so ✓
- in America there is less of a link between schools and clubs to promote participation from an early age ✓
- beyond school, in the UK there is a strong tradition of voluntary sports clubs catering for participation, which does not exist in the USA ✓
- in the UK we have organisations like Sport England that have lots of schemes with the aim of increasing participation; such an organisation does not exist in the USA ✓

> Candidate B scores 4 marks. This answer makes more correct points than marks available to ensure a maximum is achieved, but it does so in a concise manner. This answer illustrates effective exam technique as it makes several relevant points in a clearly structured way so that no time is wasted.

Candidate A

(c) The UK has put in place lots of initiatives to get more children taking part in PE as obesity is on the increase and too many are playing computer games. This means children are growing up less fit and playing less sport, particularly girls. It is different in Australia as the climate encourages lots of activity and there are lots of facilities like swimming pools. This means children in Australia are healthier than in Britain.

> Candidate A fails to score for this general descriptive account of relative participation patterns in the UK and Australia. It contains vague, irrelevant information and fails to address the initiatives and participation in school PE/sport in the countries concerned.

Candidate B

(c) Initiatives to increase participation in school PE and sport in the UK include:

- PESCCLS, which is now called PESSYP and aims to get more schoolchildren taking part in PE/sport by linking school PE departments with local sports clubs to share facilities, coaches etc ✓.
- The Youth Sport Trust has brought in TOPs, which is a series of linked programmes for children aged from 18 months to 18 years introducing sport and developing skills in a fun developmental way ✓.
- Sports colleges are secondary schools with specialist status for sport. They get extra money to provide more opportunities to do PE/sport at school ✓.
- In Australia there are also lots of schemes promoting school PE/sport such as:
  - Exemplary schools, which are prestigious schools with excellent PE teachers who are willing and able to share good practice with neighbouring schools ✓.
  - Teachers' games, which involve residential, competitive sports experiences providing network opportunities and endorsing the strong participation ethic in Australian school PE/sport ✓.
- School–club links through the 'Sports Linkage' policy involve schools and clubs sharing facilities to benefit the community ✓.

📝 Candidate B scores 6 marks. This excellent answer covers school PE/sport initiatives in the UK and in Australia. It highlights six initiatives and gives a succinct explanation of each to ensure all possible marks are gained.

Candidate A

(d) The AIS is based in Canberra while the EIS has a number of centres spread up and down the country (e.g. Loughborough). Loughborough is a specialist centre for lots of sports like cricket and netball. The EIS centres have copied the AIS as they give top-quality facilities for top-level performers to train in ✓. They also have in them lots of sport science support to develop elite performers (e.g. biomechanics and analysis of performance) ✓.

📝 Candidate A scores 2 marks. The first point made (about the difference in structure between the AIS and the EIS) is true but irrelevant. The second sentence is incorrect (neither cricket nor netball are Olympic sports developing Team GB athletes) and no marks are gained as it does not answer the question. The 2 marks are gained for the final two sentences, which illustrate knowledge of what the UK has learnt and applied from the AIS model about preparing elite-level performers.

Candidate B

(d) Team GB athletes have benefited from the UKSI being set up and containing lots of features of the AIS best-practice model such as:

- top-class coaches developing Team GB athletes to their full potential ✓
- top-class performers training in top-class facilities like specialist 50 m swimming pools at Loughborough ✓

- top-class sports medicine back-up to keep top-level performers as fit and healthy as possible ✓
- lifestyle support and advice to keep performers stress free and able to focus on training/competition ✓
- sports science research to try to give Team GB athletes an edge over their rivals in international competition ✓

Candidate B scores 5 marks. Five relevant points are given following a short introductory phrase that focuses attention on what the question demands. It often helps to spend a little time underlining/highlighting key words in the question before slightly re-wording them to form an introductory phrase for your answer. If you then address the question in clear, relevant points you are more likely to earn marks than by taking a vague, scattergun approach and making as many points as possible related to a topic.

■ ■ ■

Question 6

Individual influences on the sports performer

Explain the term 'learned helplessness' using examples from sport. As a coach, what strategies can you put in place so that performers may avoid it? (6 marks)

Candidates' answers to Question 6

Candidate A

Learned helplessness is when you don't like performing because you know you will lose ✓, e.g. you played a very good team before and lost so you think that you will fail against them again. To stop this from happening the coach should develop the performer's self-confidence ✓. This could be for one sport such as football or all sports. This is global ✓ learned helplessness.

Candidate A scores 3 marks. This is a weak answer and such limited information suggests that the candidate has run out of time. Ensure that you allocate the correct amount of time per question. While there are some credit-worthy points, there is a lack of technical terminology. The majority of this information is vague and at best would gain benefit-of-the-doubt marks.

Candidate B

Learned helplessness is when an athlete believes that no matter what they do or how hard they try they will definitely fail ✓. It could be that they think they will fail in all sports, this is known as global ✓ learned helplessness and often causes people to withdraw from sport completely. It might be that they have specific learned helplessness, which means that they think might fail in one sport or skill, e.g. I'm rubbish at tennis ✓ or I know I will miss penalties.

In order to avoid this, coaches should raise the confidence ✓ of their athletes. They could do this by setting easily achievable ✓ performance or process goals, e.g. to improve the forehand technique in tennis. The coach should praise and encourage the performer for any success. Bandura calls this verbal persuasion ✓. Attributional re-training should also be done. This is when the coach encourages the athlete to attribute failure to external reasons such as luck that may change in future fixtures.

> ✎ Candidate B scores the full 6 marks. The candidate has addressed both parts of the question and has given clear examples throughout that support the theory. This answer is clearly written using the correct technical language.

■ ■ ■

Question 7

Group dynamics of performance and audience

(a) Identify two qualities of a leader and explain how individuals become leaders. (4 marks)

(b) Explain how an athlete may be affected when performing in front of an audience. (5 marks)

Candidates' answers to Question 7

Candidate A

(a) Leaders are motivated ✓ and can motivate others. They are very skilful. Leaders can be autocratic, which means they become bossy. Or they may be democratic, which means they listen to people.

> ✎ Candidate A scores 1 mark for this limited answer. The candidate has given three qualities of a leader but gains only 1 mark. This is because the question specifies the number of qualities required, which means the examiner will only mark the first two answers given. 'Motivated and can motivate others' appear under the same point on the mark scheme, so can be credited only once. 'Skilful' will be ignored. The second part of the answer is irrelevant as the candidate has described leadership styles. Always read the question thoroughly.

Candidate B

(a) Leaders have charisma ✓. They have excellent communication ✓ skills and can empathise with others. Individuals may become prescribed or emergent leaders. Prescribed leaders are selected from outside the team ✓. For example, the ECB selected Andrew Strauss ✓. An emergent leader comes forward from within a team ✓. This might be because he or she is the best player on the team, e.g. the most skilful player on my netball team became the leader as we all respected her ✓.

> Candidate B scores 4 marks. This is an excellent answer that addresses both parts of the question successfully. The candidate has given more than two correct qualities of a leader but has reached the maximum marks available for this point. He clearly explains prescribed and emergent leaders and supports the answers with examples.

Candidate A

(b) When performing in front of a crowd the performer reverts to the dominant response ✓. This is the skill used when under pressure from being observed, e.g. a forehand ground stroke in tennis. This is caused by arousal increasing ✓. If the performer is an extrovert, he or she can cope with high arousal because he or she has naturally low levels of adrenaline detected in the RAS ✓ and needs to get excited to perform best. An introvert is the opposite.

> Candidate A scores 3 marks. This answer starts off well with clear knowledge and correct use of terminology. There are not enough points, however, to gain full marks. Always give more answers than marks available as the examiner will mark positively. Candidate A has finished off the answer disappointingly. You must fully expand your answer to gain credit at A2.

Candidate B

(b) When you are being watched, especially if significant people ✓ are in the crowd, you may become very nervous. This causes your arousal levels to rise ✓. If you are at cognitive level your performance will worsen ✓ as you are not used to performing in front of a crowd. If you are autonomous, you are used to performing with a crowd and can handle the pressure so your performance gets better ✓. Nervousness is made even worse when playing away as you don't have the homefield advantage ✓.

> Candidate B scores 5 marks although she has done the bare minimum. The examiner would have to give benefit-of-the-doubt marks as the candidate should have discussed the dominant response and its effects. The points about significant others and homefield advantage should also have been expanded. Always write comprehensive answers.

■ ■ ■

Question 8

Linear motion

(a) **Identify Newton's three laws of motion and apply each of these laws to a sporting example.** (6 marks)

(b) **In the 800 m, an athlete runs two laps of the track. What do you understand by the terms 'distance' and 'displacement'? Give values for both of these once the athlete has completed the race.** (4 marks)

Candidates' answers to Question 8

Candidate A

(a) Newton's first law of motion is where a body continues in a state of rest or motion in a straight line, unless the external forces exerted upon it change that state ✓. Newton's second law of motion is the acceleration for a body of constant mass is proportional to the force causing it and the change that takes place in the direction in which the force acts ✓. Newton's third law of motion is that for every action there is an equal and opposite reaction ✓.

> ✍ Candidate A scores 3 marks. He or she has made a common mistake — reading the first part of a question and forgetting about the second part. The candidate has failed to give any examples and lost 3 marks. Always check your work at the end of the exam to ensure these errors do not occur.

Candidate B

(a) Newton's first law of motion is that a body continues in its state of rest or motion in a straight line, unless compelled to change that state by external forces exerted upon it ✓. In football, a ball will stay on the penalty spot until it is kicked by the player. Its state of motion then changes ✓. Newton's second law of motion is that the rate of momentum of a body (or the acceleration for a body of constant mass) is proportional to the force causing it and the change that takes place in the direction in which the force acts ✓. Again in football the harder the ball is kicked, the further and faster it will go ✓. Newton's third law of motion is that for every action there is an equal and opposite reaction ✓. The harder the player pushes against the ground when jumping up to do a header the bigger the reaction from the ground ✓.

> ✍ Candidate B scores full marks. Each of Newton's three laws has been correctly identified and a relevant example given for each. The question did not specify a particular sport, so the examples could be from a range of sports or just one (as in this case). Always check what kind of example the question is asking for.

When asked for a games activity, a common mistake is to give an example from another discipline such as athletics. This would result in the loss of 3 easy marks.

Candidate A

(b) The distance the athlete runs is 800 m ✓ because she has run round the track two times. The displacement is also 800 m.

> ✐ Candidate A scores 1 mark. This answer reveals a lack of revision. The candidate has not learnt simple definitions and consequently lost 3 marks from a relatively straightforward question.

Candidate B

(b) Distance = 800 m ✓ and is the length of the path a body follows when moving from one position to another ✓. Displacement = 0 m ✓ and is the length of a straight line joining the start and finish points ✓.

> ✐ Candidate B scores 4 marks. This is an excellent 'examiner-friendly' response that answers all parts of the question in a clear, succinct manner.

■ ■ ■

Question 9

Force

(a) **Identify and draw on a free body diagram the forces acting on a 1500 m runner in the last 100 m of a race.** (4 marks)

(b) **A sprinter with a mass of 65 kg accelerated during the first 20 m of a 100 m sprint at 6.8 m s⁻². Calculate the force that is needed to achieve this (showing your calculations).** (3 marks)

Candidates' answers to Question 9

Candidate A

(a)

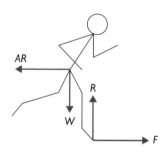

Ⓔ Candidate A scores 2 marks. This question requires knowledge of the vertical forces (weight/gravity and reaction) and the horizontal forces (air resistance and friction). The candidate has correctly identified all four forces but he has not applied friction and air resistance. In the last 100 m of the 1500 m the runner would be accelerating. This means that the friction arrow should be longer than the air resistance arrow. Make sure that you apply knowledge of these forces to the example in the question.

Candidate B

(a)

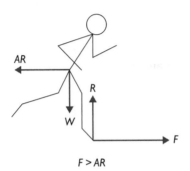

F > AR

Ⓔ Candidate B scores full marks. He has applied the free body diagram to the example given in the question and made sure that the friction arrow is longer than the air resistance arrow. This means that the runner is accelerating. When the arrows are the same size, speed is constant.

Candidate A

(b) Force = mass × acceleration ✓

$\quad\quad$ = 65 × 6.8 ✓

$\quad\quad$ = 442

Ⓔ Candidate A scores 2 marks. She has correctly identified how to calculate force but has not used the unit of measurement for her final answer, losing an easy mark.

Candidate B

(b) Force = mass × acceleration ✓

$\quad\quad$ = 65 × 6.8 ✓

$\quad\quad$ = 442 N ✓

Ⓔ Candidate B scores 3 marks. She has used the correct unit of measurement. Remember to take a calculator into your exam.

■ ■ ■

Question 10

Projectiles

(a) Identify the nature of the fluid friction force acting on a skier and describe the factors that determine its size. (3 marks)

(b) Explain what is meant by the Bernoulli principle, using the flight path of a discus to illustrate your answer. (6 marks)

Candidates' answers to Question 10

Candidate A

(a) The fluid force acting on the skier is friction because the skier is slipping down the mountain and he is going faster as the gradient gets steeper.

> Candidate A scores no marks. Friction has no effect on a skier and the rest of the answer is too vague. Questions often refer to the fluid environment of a travelling body. Remember that air resistance is the force opposing motion in air and drag is the force opposing motion in water.

Candidate B

(a) The fluid force acting on the skier is air resistance ✓. The factors that determine its size are the velocity ✓ and the body position ✓ of the skier.

> Candidate B scores 3 marks. The candidate has correctly identified the fluid friction force as air resistance and has given two factors that determine the size. Other factors include the cross-sectional area of the body and the shape/surface characteristics of the body.

Candidate A
(b)

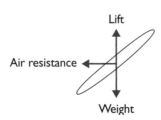

> Candidate A scores 1 mark for drawing the diagram. This is correct but too vague for any more marks. The candidate should have explained the Bernoulli principle and related it to the diagram.

Candidate B

(b) The Bernoulli principle is where air molecules exert less pressure the faster they travel ✓. This means the pressure is different on either side of a projectile ✓ such as a discus. When a discus is thrown, the air molecules have to travel further over the top ✓, which means they travel faster than those below ✓. The pressure above the discus is therefore lower than the pressure below ✓ and this causes a lift force ✓.

🖉 Candidate B scores all 6 marks. This answer correctly identifies the Bernoulli principle and relates it concisely and clearly to the flight of the discus. Marks were also available for the use of a diagram.

■ ■ ■

Question 11

Angular motion

(a) Identify and sketch the type of lever system that can be found in the ankle joint. (3 marks)

(b) Why is a diver able to perform a greater number of tucked somersaults than straight somersaults during flight? Use your understanding of the principle of conservation of angular momentum in your answer. (4 marks)

Candidates' answers to Question 11

Candidate A
(a)

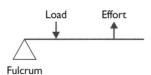

🖉 Candidate A scores 2 marks. He has drawn correctly the second-order lever system but has lost an easy mark by not identifying the order of the lever found in the ankle. Checking your answers at the end of the exam is important.

Candidate B
(a) The ankle joint is a second order lever.

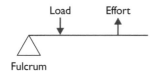

🖉 Candidate B scores full marks. He has correctly identified the lever and drawn a clear sketch. The 2 marks for the sketch were for correctly labelling the load, effort and fulcrum and for having them in the correct order.

Candidate A

(b) A diver can make her somersault go faster or slower depending on her body position. If she uses a tucked position she goes faster and in a straight position she goes slower ✓.

> 🖉 This answer scores 1 mark. It does not take into account moment of inertia or give an explanation of it. You must ensure that your revision is thorough so you are able to use all the correct technical vocabulary.

Candidate B

(b) Angular momentum = moment of inertia × angular velocity ✓. In a tucked position the diver has a low moment of inertia ✓ because her body weight is close to the axis of rotation. This means her angular velocity is high ✓ and more somersaults per flight can be performed ✓. In a straight somersault, moment of inertia is high ✓ and angular velocity is low ✓, so fewer somersaults can be performed ✓.

> 🖉 This answer scores the full 4 marks (it makes seven credit-worthy points). The answer is explained using the conservation of angular momentum and comparisons are made between the tucked and straight positions.

■ ■ ■

Question 12

Energy

(a) Describe the main energy system used by an athlete during a 400 m sprint. (6 marks)

(b) During team games, players need to manage the physiological demands of performance. The diagram below shows the average proportions of carbohydrate and fat usage during a period of exercise of increasing intensity.

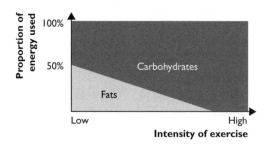

Describe what this diagram shows and explain, using your knowledge of energy systems, why this occurs. (6 marks)

Candidates' answers to Question 12

Candidate A

(a) The energy systems used by the 400m runner are the ATP-PC system and the lactic acid system ✓. The ATP-PC system is used for the first part of the race and is a simple system to use. It uses phosphocreatine as the fuel and there are no fatiguing by-products. The energy yield is 1 ATP. After 10 seconds the lactic acid system is used for the rest of the race.

> ✍ Candidate A scores 1 mark. She has named the two energy systems that are used during the 400m. However, the question asks for the *predominant* energy system. This is the lactic acid system and it should be explained.

Candidate B

(a) The main energy system is the lactic acid system ✓. This is anaerobic ✓ and glucose is broken down into pyruvic acid ✓. Two ATP molecules ✓ are formed and lactic acid is the by-product ✓. This system takes place in the sarcoplasm ✓ and the controlling enzyme is PFK ✓.

> ✍ Candidate B gains the full 6 marks. The correct energy system is identified and then explained in detail.

Candidate A

(b) At low-intensity exercise, 50% of energy comes from fats/carbohydrates ✓. This is because fats need more oxygen for their breakdown ✓ so they cannot be used anaerobically ✓.

> ✍ Candidate A scores 3 marks. There were 3 more marks available for explaining the diagram but this answer concentrated on the use of fats and missed out carbohydrates. If you are asked to comment on a diagram, marks will be available for simply saying what the diagram shows. State the obvious and discuss everything you see.

Candidate B

(b) At low-intensity exercise, 50% of energy comes from fats and 50% carbohydrates ✓. As the intensity increases, less fat and more carbohydrate is used ✓. At high intensity, carbohydrates are the only energy source ✓. At low intensity, fat and carbohydrates are broken down using oxygen ✓. Fats require more oxygen for their breakdown ✓. They are broken down in the Krebs cycle ✓. No fats can be used anaerobically ✓.

> ✍ Candidate B scores full marks. Three marks are for describing what the diagram shows and the description of the conditions and where fats and carbohydrates are broken down earn a further 3 marks. Marks were also available for mentioning glycolysis and lactate formation.

■ ■ ■

Question 13

The recovery process

At the end of a team game, players may experience EPOC. Define EPOC, give the functions of the alactacid and lactacid components of EPOC, and explain how these functions are achieved. (7 marks)

Candidates' answers to Question 13

Candidate A

EPOC stands for excess post-exercise oxygen consumption ✓. The alactacid component involves replenishing ATP and PC stores ✓ and myoglobin levels ✓. The lactacid component involves getting rid of lactic acid ✓.

> Candidate A scores 4 marks. She has explained EPOC and the functions of the alactacid and lactacid components but has not answered the last part of the question. Always check your work to make sure you haven't missed anything out.

Candidate B

EPOC is excess post-exercise oxygen consumption ✓. The alactacid component involves the restoration of ATP and PC ✓ and the resaturation of myoglobin with oxygen ✓. It takes 30 seconds for half the stores to be replenished and 3 minutes for full replenishment ✓. The lactacid component is the removal of lactic acid ✓. It is possible to get rid of lactic acid by taking in extra oxygen ✓ and oxidising it to carbon dioxide and water ✓. Some lactic acid can be converted to glycogen/glucose ✓ and protein ✓.

> Candidate B scores full marks. He has identified all areas of the question and answered each part correctly. He could have stated how much oxygen each component uses: the alactacid component uses 2–3 litres and the lactacid component uses 5–6 litres of oxygen.

■ ■ ■

Question 14

Health components of physical fitness

(a) List five structural and/or physiological reasons why the VO$_2$ max of an elite athlete may be greater than that of a fun runner. (5 marks)

(b) Circuit training is a popular method of strength training. Identify the main characteristics of circuit training and the guidelines you would follow when planning a circuit. (3 marks)

(c) Identify and explain four factors that can affect the flexibility of a performer. (4 marks)

(d) Obesity is a problem that is increasing in Western societies. What are the problems associated with childhood obesity? (5 marks)

Candidates' answers to Question 14

Candidate A

(a) The VO_2 max of elite athletes is greater because they have an increased stroke volume ✓ due to a bigger heart. They have more red blood cells ✓ and therefore more haemoglobin. They also have more capillaries ✓.

   🖉 Candidate A scores 3 marks. She has correctly identified that the question asks for only five reasons. Remember that if a question requires a number of reasons or features, the examiner will only mark that number and any subsequent answers will receive no marks. Unfortunately for Candidate A, hypertrophy of the heart means a bigger *and* stronger heart — both words have to be used to gain a mark. The points about an increase in haemoglobin levels and red blood cells were allocated the same mark.

Candidate B

(a) The VO_2 max of elite athletes is greater because they have an increased stroke volume ✓. They also have an increase in red blood cells ✓, and the number of mitochondria ✓. OBLA levels are higher ✓ and they have an increase in their glycogen and triglyceride stores ✓.

   🖉 Candidate B scores 5 marks. She has mentioned five different areas, so avoiding repetition of marks. Marks would have been awarded for bradycardia, increase in maximum minute ventilation, improved diffusion rates, increases in the elasticity of arterial walls and slow-twitch hypertrophy.

Candidate A

(b) Circuit training is designed to improve muscular endurance ✓. It consists of small stations of exercises such as press-ups and running activities ✓.

   🖉 Candidate A scores 2 marks. A common mistake is to answer the question in a rush and forget the second part. This answer misses out the guidelines. Always check to ensure you have answered all parts of a question.

Candidate B

(b) Circuit training improves muscular endurance ✓. It consists of different stations of exercises such as sit-ups as well as running activities ✓. A circuit is continuous so it is important to rotate the muscle groups ✓ to avoid fatigue and make sure the age and fitness of the group ✓ is taken into account.

📝 This candidate scores full marks. She has correctly identified both the characteristics and the guidelines associated with circuit training.

Candidate A

(c) Flexibility can be affected by how old you are, how much training you do, gender and whether or not you do a warm-up.

📝 Candidate A fails to score. Although he has identified four factors that can affect flexibility, he has not explained these factors and has lost easy marks.

Candidate B

(c) Flexibility can be affected by a person's age: the older you are the less flexible you are ✓. Training can also have an effect. Regular flexibility training keeps joints more mobile ✓. The type of joint is also important, hinge joints only allow flexion and extension whereas ball-and-socket joints have a much greater range of movement ✓. A warm-up also increases flexibility as it increases the temperature of the surrounding muscle and connective tissue ✓.

📝 Candidate B scores maximum marks. He has correctly identified and explained four factors that affect flexibility. Other answers could have included the structure of a joint, for example the joint cavity of the shoulder is much shallower and the ligaments looser than that of the hip, which allows for greater flexibility.

Candidate A

(d) Being obese means you are overweight and this leads to lots of problems, for example heart disease at a young age ✓ and also diabetes ✓. Cholesterol builds up in the arteries and this causes problems for blood flow.

📝 Candidate A scores 2 marks. This question is worth 5 marks so at the very least there should be five answers. Cholesterol levels do build up but more detail is needed: it is levels of LDL cholesterol that are high. When a question does not ask for a specific number of reasons, always give more answers than the mark allocation.

Candidate B

(d) An obese person has high fat and sugar levels in his body and this can lead to high blood pressure ✓, diabetes ✓ and premature heart disease ✓. Due to the excess weight he may also have back pain ✓ and joint damage ✓.

📝 This answer scores full marks. The candidate has looked at the mark allocation and given the correct number of answers. She could have given more just to make sure of full marks, in case one answer was incorrect. Marks would have been awarded for high levels of LDL cholesterol and limitations in mobility or flexibility.

■ ■ ■

Question 15

Training and ergogenic aids

(a) **When planning a training programme, periodisation is important. Explain what is meant by this term.** (4 marks)

(b) **Name two illegal ergogenic aids that may be of benefit to an endurance performer, explaining how they can help performance and highlighting any possible side effects.** (6 marks)

(c) **Explain the importance of an ice bath as a recovery/cooling aid for an elite performer.** (3 marks)

Candidates' answers to Question 15

Candidate A
(a) Periodisation is when the training programme is split into stages ✓. It contains the macrocycle, mesocycle and microcycles ✓.

> 🖉 Candidate A scores 2 marks. He has correctly identified the meaning of periodisation and the names of the stages. However, the question asks for an explanation. If the candidate had explained what each of these cycles meant, he would have gained full marks.

Candidate B
(a) Periodisation is when the training year is divided up into periods or stages ✓. The macrocycle is the long-term goal, for example getting a personal best time ✓. The mesocycle is period of training lasting about a month where a particular aspect of the programme is focused on ✓. The microcycle is a description of a week's training sessions ✓.

> 🖉 Candidate B scores full marks. Other marks would have been awarded for mentioning pre-season training, allowing for out-of-season recovery and for peaking or tapering.

Candidate A
(b) HGH ✓ is an artificially produced hormone that is used to increase muscle mass ✓. Prolonged use can lead to heart and nerve disease ✓. Steroids also produce muscle growth but lead to acne and liver or heart disease.

> 🖉 Candidate A scores 3 marks. The question asks for two illegal aids that would be useful to an endurance performer. Steroids are illegal but they are used mainly by power athletes, so the candidate has lost 3 marks by writing about the wrong aid. The specification requires you to know which type of performer uses which aids, so check the question to see which performer you need to discuss.

Candidate B

(b) HGH ✓ is used by endurance athletes to increase muscle mass ✓ and cause a decrease in body fat ✓. It can cause heart and nerve disease ✓, glucose intolerance and a high level of blood fats ✓. Rh-EPO ✓ is also used. It is a hormone that can be artificially made to increase the oxygen-carrying capacity of the blood ✓. It can, however, result in blood clotting and strokes ✓.

Candidate B scores full marks. She has correctly chosen two aids for an endurance performer and explained what they are, how they help performance and highlighted the side effects associated with them. Other aids the candidate could have discussed are gene doping and blood doping.

Candidate A

(c) An ice bath is good because it cools the muscles down and helps them to recover quicker. However it sounds very painful and I do not think I would like to try one.

Candidate A scores no marks. It is obvious the candidate has not revised this area because there is no detail in the answer.

Candidate B

(c) At the end of strenuous training sessions it is important for an elite performer to take an ice bath. He needs to stay in an ice bath for 5 to 10 minutes ✓. This is because the cold causes the blood vessels to tighten and drains the blood out of the legs ✓. When he leaves the bath his legs fill up with new blood containing oxygen ✓. The blood that leaves the legs takes away with it the lactic acid that has built up during the weight training session ✓.

This is an excellent answer with all the required detail, scoring full marks.